Wall Pilates Power

A Woman's Guide to Strength and Grace

Introduction

There is a sanctuary where grace and power meet, where the path to self-discovery energizes and transforms among the tumult and pressures of contemporary life that pull us in all directions. Thank you for visiting "Wall Pilates Power: A Woman's Guide to Strength and Grace."

A comprehensive approach to well-being is becoming increasingly important as we manage the obstacles of everyday life. "Wall Pilates Power" is more than simply a workout manual; it's an empowering ally on your path to developing physical strength and emotional peace. Taking inspiration from the concepts of Pilates and cleverly modified to work with a wall as support, this book is meant primarily for women looking for a straightforward, step-by-step approach to building strength, flexibility, and mindfulness.

Let's examine the fundamentals of Wall Pilates first before delving into the methods and details that will completely transform how you interact with your body. This technique, which has its roots in Joseph Pilates's philosophy, is well known for its capacity to unite the mind, body, and soul. Adding the wall aspect opens up possibilities by combining the wall's structure and support with the fundamental Pilates concepts.

This book is more than simply a collection of exercises; it's a whole manual that takes you through the background and tenets of Pilates, highlights the many advantages specifically designed for women and helps you set up a place specifically for your Wall Pilates practice. As you go through each chapter, you will learn about posture and spine alignment, flexibility improvement, upper body and arm toning, lower body concentration, core strengthening, and advanced methods that will push and improve your physical capabilities.

"Wall Pilates Power" is designed for everyone starting in the Pilates world or for seasoned practitioners looking to add something new to their routine. Accept the challenge, acknowledge your accomplishments, and enjoy the process of molding your body and mind into the shape you want.

Prepare to reach your full potential, achieve equilibrium in your movements, and become the formidable combination of elegance and strength. Start the trip now.

Chapter 1: Introduction to Wall Pilates

1.1: History and Principles of Pilates

The name Joseph Pilates reverberates with the resonance of creativity and thoughtful movement throughout the quiet hallways of fitness history. Pilates originated in the early 20th century when German gymnast Joseph Pilates created a groundbreaking method of training that goes beyond just physical effort. Pilates's history is more than simply a list of exercises; it's a tale of change, resiliency, and the persistent conviction that the mind and body are inextricably linked.

The Genesis: The Unveiled Vision of Joseph Pilates

Joseph Pilates was born in Mönchengladbach, Germany, in 1883. During his early years, he had to deal with the complex reality of fragile health. He was motivated to go beyond these physical constraints, so he immersed himself in a wide range of fitness practices, taking cues from ancient Greek and Roman workout routines and gymnastics, yoga, and martial arts—the roots of what we know as this diverse blending of influences sowed Pilates.

Early in the 1920s, Joseph Pilates and his wife Clara relocated to the US and opened a studio in New York City. The Pilates technique began with a couple committed to rehabilitation; they worked with dancers and athletes to improve performance and help them recover from injuries. Over time, the Pilates technique developed into a whole system of mental and physical fitness, moving beyond the field of rehabilitation.

Time-Transcending Principles: The Fundamentals of Pilates

A series of tenets that are the cornerstone of Pilates' philosophy are located at its core. These carefully considered ideas, developed by Joseph Pilates, emphasize a comprehensive approach to well-being and go beyond physical activities.

1. Centering:

The center of Pilates is the core, often known as the powerhouse. By activating the deep abdominal, lower back, hip, and buttock muscles, one may establish a solid and steady core from which all other motions originate. This approach develops a concentrated and focused mind and strengthens the physical core.

2. Control:

Pilates is known for its accuracy and control. Each action is performed with purpose and awareness, guaranteeing that the muscles are used throughout the full range of motion. This focus on control encourages awareness and keeps the body from experiencing needless stress.

3. Precision:

In Pilates, more is needed regarding quality. Every action is performed precisely, requiring a high awareness of muscle activation and body alignment. A healthy and well-sculpted body is developed via the precision of Pilates.

4. Mean Mindfulness:

A fundamental component of Pilates is the mind-body connection. To concentrate, one must train one's mind to focus on the work at hand and practice awareness in their movements. By focusing on the breath and movement, practitioners raise their level of awareness generally and get the most out of the exercises.

5. Breath:

According to Joseph Pilates, the breath is the force behind the movement. In Pilates, the breath is deep, regulated, and timed to fit each movement. Breathing correctly improves the mind-body connection, increases energy flow, and oxygenates the body.

6. Progress:

The fluidity, smoothness, and continuity of Pilates exercises are intended. Flow facilitates the smooth integration of strength and flexibility by encouraging elegant transitions between exercises. Pilates's rhythmic flow encourages fluidity in both movement and mind.

Collectively referred to as the "Pilates Principles," these ideas stand the test of time and serve as the foundation for every Pilates practice. They provide a framework that influences everyday life and directs physical activity, encouraging a conscious and well-rounded way of living.

Today's Pilates: An Eternal Legacy

It is clear from studying the foundations and history of Pilates that its influence goes far beyond the boundaries of exercise programs. Pilates is evidence of the transforming potential of conscious movement—a journey that combines the historical and the modern, the cerebral and the physical. The teachings of Joseph Pilates are still relevant in a world where people are continuously looking for holistic well-being. They encourage people to go on a path of self-discovery, resilience, and the unwavering quest for balance.

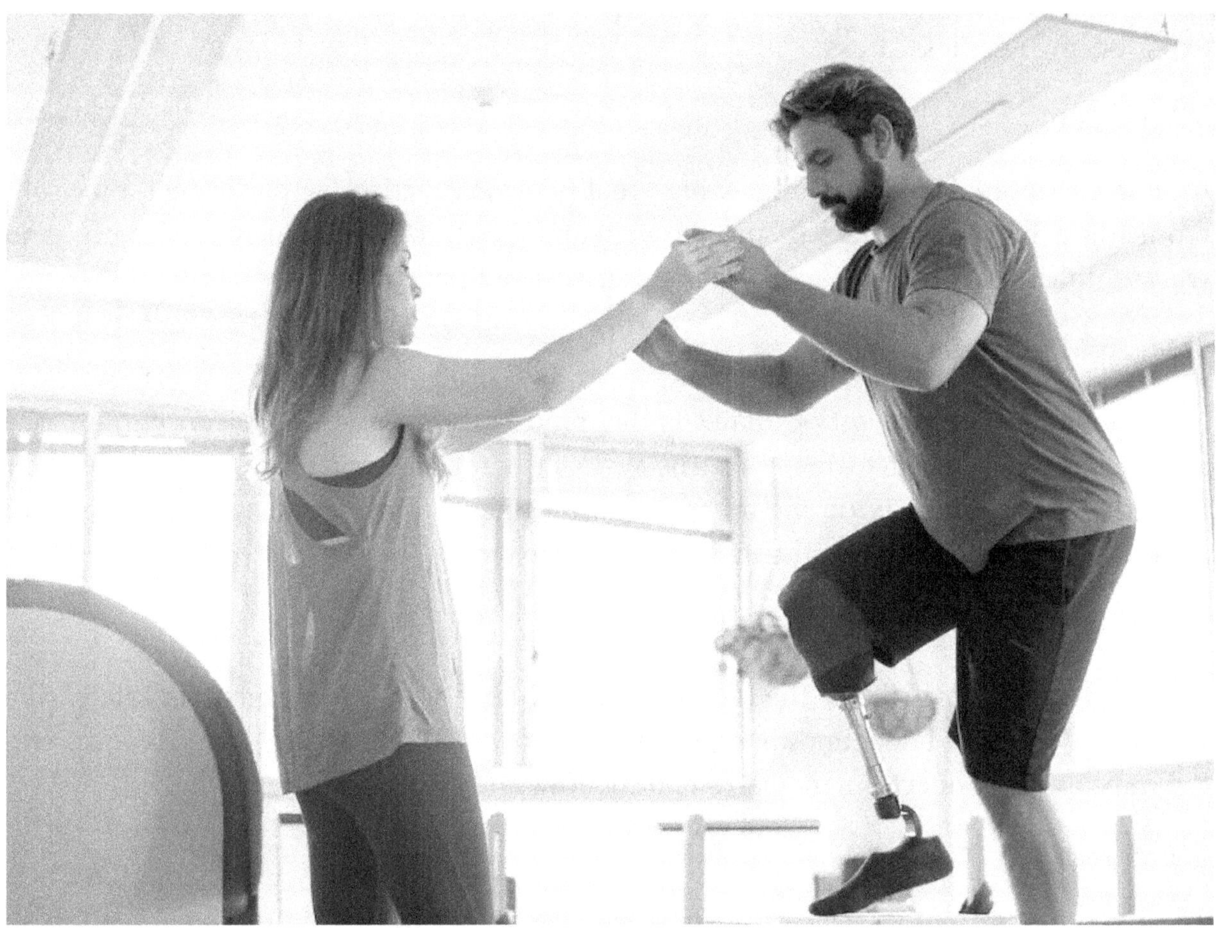

1.2: Benefits of Wall Pilates for Women

Within the fitness industry, where fads come and go, Wall Pilates is a shining example of transforming exercise designed to support women on their path to overall wellness. Strength, elegance, and conscious movement are combined in Wall Pilates, a workout method that goes beyond traditional notions of what constitutes physical fitness. Let's explore the many advantages that Wall Pilates offers to women, as it shapes their bodies and strengthens the connection between their minds and bodies.

1. Selected Core Capabilities:

The foundation of Wall Pilates focuses on core strength, which extends beyond the muscles on the surface. Traditional Pilates exercises get depth from integrating the wall, which calls for a greater engagement of the back, pelvic, and abdominal muscles. This focused core practice helps women develop better posture, stability, and a solid foundation for everyday tasks and toning their midsections.

2. Flexibility and Availability:

Wall Pilates is an excellent option for women of all fitness levels since it provides a flexible and approachable training method. The wall offers support and stability, enabling adjustments and progressive advancement, whether you are a novice wishing to introduce yourself to Pilates or an experienced practitioner looking to spice up your practice. Wall Pilates is inclusive because it can be customized to meet the requirements of anyone with a range of abilities.

3. Increased Range of Motion and Flexibility:

Pilates exercises that use the wall allow for controlled stretches and extensions, improving flexibility and increasing range of motion. This feature is especially beneficial for women since it increases joint mobility, lowers the chance of injury, and promotes fluidity in movement. Women can explore and realize their bodies' most significant potential via wall Pilates.

4. Mind-Body Connection for Empowerment:

Fundamentally, Pilates is a conscious exercise that emphasizes the mind-body connection. In this path of self-determination, the wall turns into a reliable friend, offering encouragement and a focal point. Women who do Wall Pilates have enhanced body awareness, mindfulness during movement, and a deep understanding of how mental concentration improves physical performance. Beyond the gym, this mind-body connection influences everyday life with a feeling of presence and purpose.

5. Back Health and Postural Alignment:

Modern sedentary lives often lead to postural abnormalities, which is where Wall Pilates comes into play as a remedial tool. The exercises improve alignment, strengthen the muscles supporting the spine, and increase postural awareness. Wall Pilates becomes a haven for promoting robust and well-supported posture, easing pain, and nourishing back health for women struggling with extended sitting or desk employment.

6. Effective and Safe Exercise for Expectant and New Mothers:

Wall Pilates is a safe and helpful option for women in the prenatal and postpartum stages because of its versatility. Because the wall offers support, workouts may be adjusted to meet the unique requirements and difficulties of pregnancy and the healing process after giving birth. Doing Wall Pilates helps support the body's natural changes during these stages while preserving strength and stability.

7. Strengthening and Toning without Bulking:

Wall Pilates is the perfect option for ladies who want to gain strength and tone without worrying about bulking up. The shaping effect is achieved without encouraging excessive muscular growth because of the deliberate motions, focus on lengthening muscles and wall integration. This is a feature that many women who value a defined body and lean, functional strength find appealing.

8. Mindful Relaxation and Stress Reduction:

In addition to its physical advantages, Wall Pilates provides a calm environment for conscious relaxation and stress alleviation. An attentive breathwork combined with the rhythmic flow of motions produces a contemplative experience. Women find comfort in the combination of breath and movement, which enables them to relax, let go of stress, and develop a feeling of calmness despite the rigors of everyday life.

9. Empowerment and Community:

Engaging in Wall Pilates often goes beyond solitary exercises, promoting empowerment and camaraderie among female participants. Women may encourage and inspire one another in a friendly atmosphere created by group courses or shared experiences. Wall Pilates's community component enriches the road toward general well-being by fostering relationships beyond the studio's doors.

10. Empowerment and Wellness Throughout Life:

Overall, Wall Pilates has several advantages for women beyond the gym. It turns into a route to empowerment and long-term well-being. Core strength, flexibility, mindfulness, and community—values developed through Wall Pilates—become pillars in women's lives, influencing decisions, encouraging resilience, and fostering an all-encompassing feeling of well-being well-being.

Wall Pilates stands out as a melodic note in the symphony of workout methods, speaking to women's particular demands and goals. It is an invitation to uncover the innate elegance, power, and resiliency that characterize every woman; it is more than just a set of moves. Women who practice Wall Pilates set out on a path of self-discovery, discovering empowerment in each deliberate movement, deliberate breath, and the bonds formed between the body and mind.

1.3: Setting Up Your Wall Pilates Space

An essential factor in achieving overall well-being is the setting in which we exercise. It's not enough to arrange equipment in a designated area for your Wall Pilates practice; you must also create an environment that fosters attention, intention, and a feeling of personal sanctuary. Explore the subtleties of designing your own Wall Pilates sanctuary, where movement and environment work in unison to enhance your practice.

1. Choosing the Ideal Area:

The first step in setting up a supportive atmosphere for your Wall Pilates practice is selecting the appropriate area. Choose a space with plenty of natural light since this improves the atmosphere and gives it a lively feel. To enable free mobility, make sure the area is well-ventilated and clutter-free. Consider designating a particular area, such as a corner, where you may create a regular practice schedule.

2. Tidying Up the Canvas:

First, clean the canvas and organize your room before adding Pilates equipment. Take out anything extra that might obstruct your path or cause diversions. In addition to improving safety, a neat and orderly environment helps people feel at ease and concentrate better. Please consider the area a blank canvas ready to be painted with the strokes of your Pilates practice as you clean it.

3. Selecting the Wall:

Without question, the wall itself is the defining feature of Wall Pilates. Choose a wall for your practice that is structurally solid and clear of obstructions. The ideal fence is plain and devoid of any fittings or projecting components. Your anchor will be this wall, providing you stability and support while you do different exercises. Consider the wall's measurements to ensure you have enough room to walk about and that the wall can support the whole length of your mat.

4. Purchasing Necessary Equipment:

Although Wall Pilates only sometimes needs a little equipment, having a few basics might help you improve. Invest in a premium Pilates mat to provide your activities with a pleasant surface. A stability ball and resistance bands are other valuable additions to your exercise regimen that may provide challenge and variation. To ensure a well-rounded and productive practice, ensure the equipment you choose aligns with your fitness level and objectives.

5. Establishing a Harmonious Environment:

Add components to your Wall Pilates area that help create a peaceful environment. Think about using plants to add natural elements and create a calm background. Ambient, soft lighting may improve the atmosphere and foster calm. Focus points may be motivated by adding personal touches like motivational slogans or pictures. Make the environment what you want it to be so you want to return repeatedly.

6. Creating Adequate Lighting:

An important factor in determining the atmosphere of your Wall Pilates practice is lighting. If natural light isn't unavailable, use soft, diffused artificial lighting instead. It might be distracting to have harsh or glaring lighting, so try to have a soft glow that fills the room. Consider using adjustable lighting to create a customized atmosphere that can accommodate various workouts and emotions.

7. Assuring Sufficient Airflow:

A pleasant and stimulating Pilates practice requires a well-ventilated area. Ensure you have enough ventilation by opening windows or utilizing fans, mainly while doing more vigorous workouts. In addition to being physically comforting, fresh air improves mental clarity and creates an atmosphere that allows you to engage in the focused movements of Wall Pilates completely.

8. Mirror Surface Configuration:

Integrating a reflective surface into your wall Pilates studios is sound for motivational and practical reasons. Mirrors provide visual feedback during workouts to assess your alignment and form. They also give the area an air of openness, which enlarges the room and strengthens the connection between your body and mind. Try to arrange the mirror to see yourself from several perspectives.

9. Setting Up Your Gear:

A smooth practice is facilitated by having your Pilates equipment organized effectively. As you prepare your mat for use, ensure it's unrolled and in its designated spot. Maintain the organization and accessibility of any additional equipment, such as stability balls and resistance bands. Maintaining a tidy workspace simplifies your routine and encourages self-control and dedication.

10. Customizing Your Environment:

Add things that speak to your goals and personality to your Wall Pilates room. Personalization gives your practice space a unique touch, whether through inspirational sayings, cherished photos, or a beloved color scheme. Think about making a vision board that summarizes your health objectives and acts as a visual guide for your path.

When you begin organizing your Wall Pilates studio, remember that it is a living, breathing representation of your dedication to health and wellness. Adjust the surroundings to suit your tastes so it may serve as a place of inspiration and renewal. Your Wall Pilates retreat transforms from a physical area into a paradise where self-discovery, mindfulness, and movement flow together. Enter this area purposefully, and use it as a blank canvas to create the masterpiece on your path toward well-being.

1.4: Safety Tips and Body Awareness

Starting a Wall Pilates adventure is a thrilling way to explore your strength, flexibility, and awareness of movement. However, safety always comes first when trying to achieve well-being well-being. Comprehending the subtleties of your body and implementing essential safety precautions guarantee a harmonious practice that not only produces physical advantages but also cultivates a profound awareness of your body. Let's explore the fundamental safety guidelines and the practice of developing body awareness in wall Pilates.

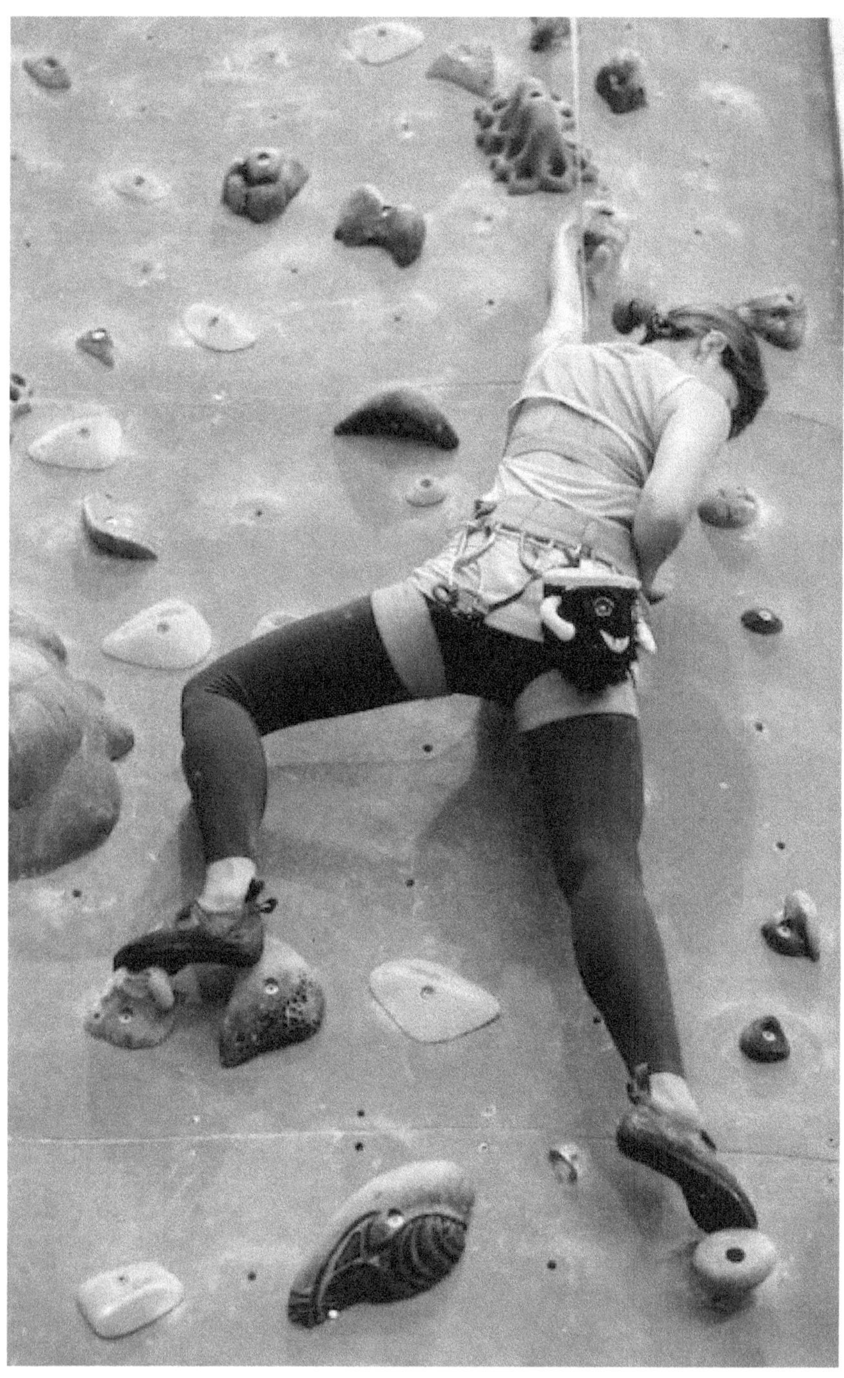

1. Start with a Contemplative Warm-Up:

Warming up mindfully before a Wall Pilates session helps your body get ready for the dynamic movements that will come next. Take part in mild activities that help open your joints, improve blood flow, and work your major muscle groups. Pay close attention to the regions like the shoulders, hips, and core that will be performed throughout the session. In addition to lowering your chance of injury, warming up prepares your body for maximum performance.

2. Pay Attention to Your Body:

The foundation of a secure and successful Wall Pilates practice is body awareness. Develop the skill of listening to your body and becoming aware of its signs and messages. When you feel strain, pain, or discomfort while exercising, stop and evaluate. Respecting the boundaries that your body sends forth is a sign of self-care. Aim for equilibrium between challenging yourself and honoring your body's unique requirements.

3. Use Correct Form:

Proper form is an essential component of Wall Pilates safety, not merely a cosmetic one. Every exercise is designed to target specific muscles and encourage balanced gait patterns. Put more emphasis on perfecting form than intensity, ensuring that your body is aligned and supported throughout every exercise. Use mirrors or recorded videos to check your form and make any corrections.

4. Accomplish Over Time:

Wall Pilates is a discipline where mastery is attained via steady practice. Refrain from jumping into more difficult activities without building a solid foundation. After mastering the fundamentals, please work on more intricate versions. Not only does this reduce the chance of damage, but it also gives your body time to adjust and gradually gain strength.

5. Make Sensible Use of Wall Support:

In Wall Pilates, the wall is a steady partner, providing stability and support. But it's crucial to make sensible use of this assistance. The wall should supplement your practice rather than take the place of your muscles; it is a guide, not a crutch. Even while using the wall for support, keep your muscles engaged and make sure your motions are deliberate and controlled.

6. Modify Intensity Depending on Your Degree of Fitness:

Because Pilates can be adjusted to meet different fitness levels, it may be challenging for seasoned practitioners and accessible to novices. Adjust the rigor of your routine to suit your present fitness level and ability. Rise the difficulty gradually as your skill and strength increase. By ensuring a sustainable and gradual path, this strategy guards against injury and overexertion.

7. Conscious Inhalation:

Pilates follows the breath, and practicing conscious breathing increases safety and effectiveness. Breathe in unison with each action, using deliberate intakes and releases to maintain the exercises' natural flow. In addition to improving bodily oxygenation, mindful breathing fosters a stronger mind-body connection that aids in concentration and relaxation.

8. Establish a Sturdy Pilates Area:

The steadiness of your Pilates area influences your practice's safety. Ensure your mat is securely in place and avoid slick surfaces. Ensure that any supplementary equipment, such as stability balls or resistance bands, is securely attached to prevent mishaps. You can move confidently in a steady practice setting because you know that your surroundings will help, not impede, your motions.

9. Make Use of Regular Rest Periods:

Even though there is a lot of appeal to moving nonstop, taking frequent breaks is essential to avoiding weariness and preserving peak performance. Weariness may impair form and raise the possibility of becoming hurt. When your body tells you it's tired, pay attention to those signals, take little pauses, and return to your practice with enthusiasm and concentration.

10. Always Remain Hydrated and Fed:

Maintaining a healthy diet and hydration regimen is essential to a safe and productive Wall Pilates practice. Ensure you drink enough water before, during, and after your workout. Consider including a well-balanced snack to give your body the energy it needs before exercise — sufficient hydration and nutrition support general well-being and physical performance.

11. Speak with an Expert:

Speaking with a fitness expert or healthcare provider if you're new to Pilates or have any underlying health issues is a good idea. They may advise based on your particular requirements, ensuring that your Wall Pilates routine complements your unique health profile. Expert advice is essential for those managing post-injury rehabilitation or specific medical issues.

Your trusty companions in the rhythmic dance of Wall Pilates are safety and body awareness. Accept the path with awareness, understanding that Pilates is about more than just physical change — it's about developing a deep connection with your body. Your Wall Pilates practice becomes a haven of self-discovery, resilience, and the ageless quest for overall well-being by including these safety guidelines and fostering body awareness.

1.5: Basic Wall Pilates Stance and Posture

The fundamentals of stance and posture set the stage for an enchanted voyage into Wall Pilates, where elegance and power collide. The canvas that the art of Pilates is created upon is our body alignment. Fundamental Wall Exercises Posture and stance are the foundation of the whole practice; they are not only the first stages. Let's explore the nuances of this core principle, where body and mind synchronization starts a healing process leading to increased strength, flexibility, and overall health.

1. Based on Conscious Alignment:

Mindful alignment is the foundation of Basic Wall Pilates Stance & Posture. Take a tall stance with your feet hip-width apart and firmly planted on the ground. By equally distributing your weight across both feet, you may develop stability. Stretch your spine by visualizing a cord pulling you upward from the top of your head. Every Pilates movement is built on this conscious alignment, which also serves as a representation of the mindful philosophy that underpins Pilates.

2. Activating the Central:

The center of strength and stability in Pilates is the core, often called the powerhouse. Bring your navel slightly toward your spine to activate your core as you take the Basic Wall Pilates Stance. By creating a link between the deep abdominal muscles and the spine, this activation creates a solid base for movement. Core engagement aims to develop a soft, encouraging engagement that flows with every action rather than becoming stiff.

3. Down and Back Shoulders:

In Wall Pilates, how the shoulders are positioned is crucial to keeping the chest open and promoting healthy breathing. Your chest will naturally expand as you roll your shoulders back and forth. In addition to improving posture, this alignment helps to release stress in the upper back and neck. It should feel like your chest is opening up and more expansive over your collarbones.

4. Slack Jaw and Neck:

It's crucial to balance exertion and rest while aiming for strength. Keep your mouth and neck loose, and don't hold yourself back. In addition to making a person feel more comfortable overall, a relaxed neck guarantees that the core and the targeted muscle groups are the center of attention throughout every exercise. Visualize your neck gently stretching outward while keeping your posture neutral and without hunching over or leaning back.

5. Soft Knees and Proper Hip Alignment:

In Basic Wall Pilates, bending the knees helps create a dynamic but secure stance. Keep your knees slightly bent instead of locking them. In addition to protecting the joints, this softening promotes a seamless transition between the lower body and the core. Ensure your shoulders and hips are in line; do not rotate or tilt. The hips link the upper and lower bodies, and a smooth range of motion depends on their alignment.

6. Grounding With Your Foot:

In Wall Pilates, your feet serve as the anchors that hold you to the ground. Spread your toes for more stability as the earth touches your feet. Keep this grounding going as you do different exercises, and let it be your point of reference for movement and balance. Grounded at the core of every activity, the awareness of your feet provides a tangible link to the here and now.

7. Putting a Plumb Line on Display:

An effective technique to keep your body aligned is to picture a plumb line passing through it. Picture this imaginary line going through your shoulders, hips, knees, ankles, and head. Maintaining a straight body with no deviations or misalignments is the aim. You may use this imagery as a guide to help you maintain balance and symmetry in your basic wall stance during Pilates.

8. Breathe In Mindfully:

The living energy that gives each Pilates action vigor is breath. In the Pilates Basic Wall Stance, concentrate on developing an awareness of your breathing rhythm. Exhale completely through pursed lips after taking a big breath through your nose and stretching your rib cage. Breathing should be regular and continuous to enhance core activation and improve general body awareness. You connect to the present moment with each breath, which turns into a moving dance.

9. Retaining an Enthusiastic Presence

The Basic Wall Pilates Stance is dynamic, yet it gives off an air of elegance and steadiness. Adopt a forceful demeanor in this base alignment. Allow the posture to change as you go through the exercises to meet the needs of each one. The dynamic presence makes the fluid transition between workouts possible, which guarantees that your body stays sensitive and involved.

10. Combining All Exercises:

The Basic Wall Pilates Stance is an ongoing element integrated into each exercise rather than a ritual to be performed at the start and finish of your practice. Alignment, activating the core, and taking deliberate breaths are the same whether you're working on your upper body, lower body, or both. Integration guarantees that every detail of your practice embodies the Basic Wall Pilates Stance principles.

As you connect yourself with the timeless principles that characterize the Pilates philosophy, you do more than establish a stance as you stand in the Basic Wall Pilates Stance. This basic pose serves as the starting point for a journey where elegance and power come together, and every movement is like a brushstroke on the canvas of your well-being. The complexity of Pilates, an artistic blend of attention, accuracy, and the liberating realization of your body's innate strength, is concealed in the simplicity of the stance.

1.6: Breathing Techniques in Wall Pilates

The breath appears as a quiet director, arranging the movement symphony in the rhythmic dance of Wall Pilates, where elegance and power blend. The breathing exercises used in Wall Pilates go beyond the essential act of breathing in and out; they develop into a living force that nourishes, energizes, and unites the body and mind. We set out on a journey where every breath is a brushstroke, painting the canvas of our well-being as we dig into the nuances of Pilates breathing.

1. The Breath Principle of Pilates:

The fundamental relationship between breath and movement lies at the heart of the Pilates concept. According to Joseph Pilates, breathing drives all exercise, establishing a mutually beneficial interaction between the respiratory system and muscle activation. The Pilates Principle of Breath is central to Wall Pilates, converting every exercise into a conscious investigation of the breath's tremendous impact on total vitality, strength, and stability.

2. Breathing Diaphragmatically

Diaphragmatic breathing is the foundation of Pilates breathing exercises. With this technique, the diaphragm, the primary breathing muscle, is deliberately and wholly engaged. Breathe deeply through your nose to expand your lungs and let the diaphragm drop. Bring your navel toward your spine to completely release the air and exhale through pursed lips. In addition to providing the body with oxygen, diaphragmatic breathing engages the deep core muscles, which helps to provide a solid base for Pilates exercises.

3. Breathing in a Regular Rhythm:

Breath creates a rhythmic flow in Wall Pilates, dictating the movement speed. Exhaling goes hand in hand with contraction and movement execution, whilst inhaling starts expansion and preparation. Breath and movement in unison produce a smooth, flowing rhythm that improves the efficacy and efficiency of every workout. The breath takes on the role of a dancing partner, guiding and helping the body into each complex stretch and position.

4. Expansion of the Ribcage:

Pilates breathing promotes the maximum use of lung capacity by encouraging an expansive movement of the rib cage. Imagine the ribs spreading out to the back and laterally as you inhale, giving your chest a wider appearance. This comprehensive breathing technique increases the amount of oxygen taken in while lengthening the spine and activating the back muscles. The rib cage transforms into a three-dimensional space that envelops the breath in every direction.

5. Activating the Abdominal Transverse:

Pilates's signature technique is the synchronization of breathing with specific muscles. The deepest layer of the abdominal muscles, the transverse abdominis, is essential in Wall Pilates. When you release the breath, concentrate on activating the transverse abdominis by pulling the navel toward the spine. This activation creates a harmonic interaction between deep abdominal engagement and controlled exhalation, strengthening core stability while promoting a conscious connection with the breath.

6. Fostering Body-Mind Awareness:

In Wall Pilates, breathing becomes a tool for developing body-mind awareness. A strong connection with the present moment is fostered by paying conscious attention to each breath in and out. The breath acts as a guide by guiding attention to the subtleties of movement, alignment, and muscle activation. A mindful breathing technique that cultivates mind-body awareness turns Pilates into a contemplative path of self-knowledge and empowerment.

7. Refraining from Holding Your Breath:

The avoidance of breath-holding is one of the fundamentals of Pilates breathing. Throughout the session, you are urged to breathe continuously and rhythmically. Breathing too forcefully causes stress, impairs smooth motion, and stops oxygen from reaching the muscles. Accept breathing in a rhythmic, continuous pattern; let the breath be your constant partner, supporting and enhancing every action.

8. Breathing as a Grounding Mechanism:

The breath becomes a stabilizing and directing factor in Wall Pilates exercises. Please take a minute to focus on yourself via deliberate breathing before beginning any workout. Breathe out completely, letting go of any stress and outside distractions, then inhale deeply to bring energy into the body. This centring breath creates a focused and attentive framework for the ensuing movements by connecting the mind and body.

9. Overcoming Difficulties:

With difficulties that increase in severity, the breath becomes a steady partner in Wall Pilates movements. Keep your breathing consistent and controlled while doing more challenging exercises or holds. Accept the breath as a source of resiliency and use it to help you stay composed and in control during difficult times. In addition to enhancing physical performance, breathing through difficulties builds mental toughness.

10. Conscientious Breathing After Exercise:

After your Wall Pilates practice, use focused breathing to ease into a post-exercise period. Take a few minutes to practice mindful, easy breathing to help your body find balance again. This focused breathing after a workout transitions between the intensity of the effort and the gradual return to a grounded, centered state.

The breath is the unseen thread that connects strength, flexibility, and awareness in the intricate tapestry of Wall Pilates. The breathing exercises used in Wall Pilates are an art form that goes beyond simple physical exercise and includes a journey towards self-awareness and empowerment. Remember that breath is more than the air entering your lungs as you breathe through each action; it is life itself coursing through you, assisting you in reaching a harmonious union of body and soul.

1.7: Understanding Your Body's Limits

The path to power and elegance in the alluring world of Wall Pilates is shown in how exercises are performed and in the subtle awareness of one's body. Recognizing your body's limitations is essential to a secure and efficient Wall Pilates practice. It invites a thorough examination of one's talents, possible obstacles, and the discernment to strike a careful balance between advancement and self-care. It goes beyond simple geographical limitations.

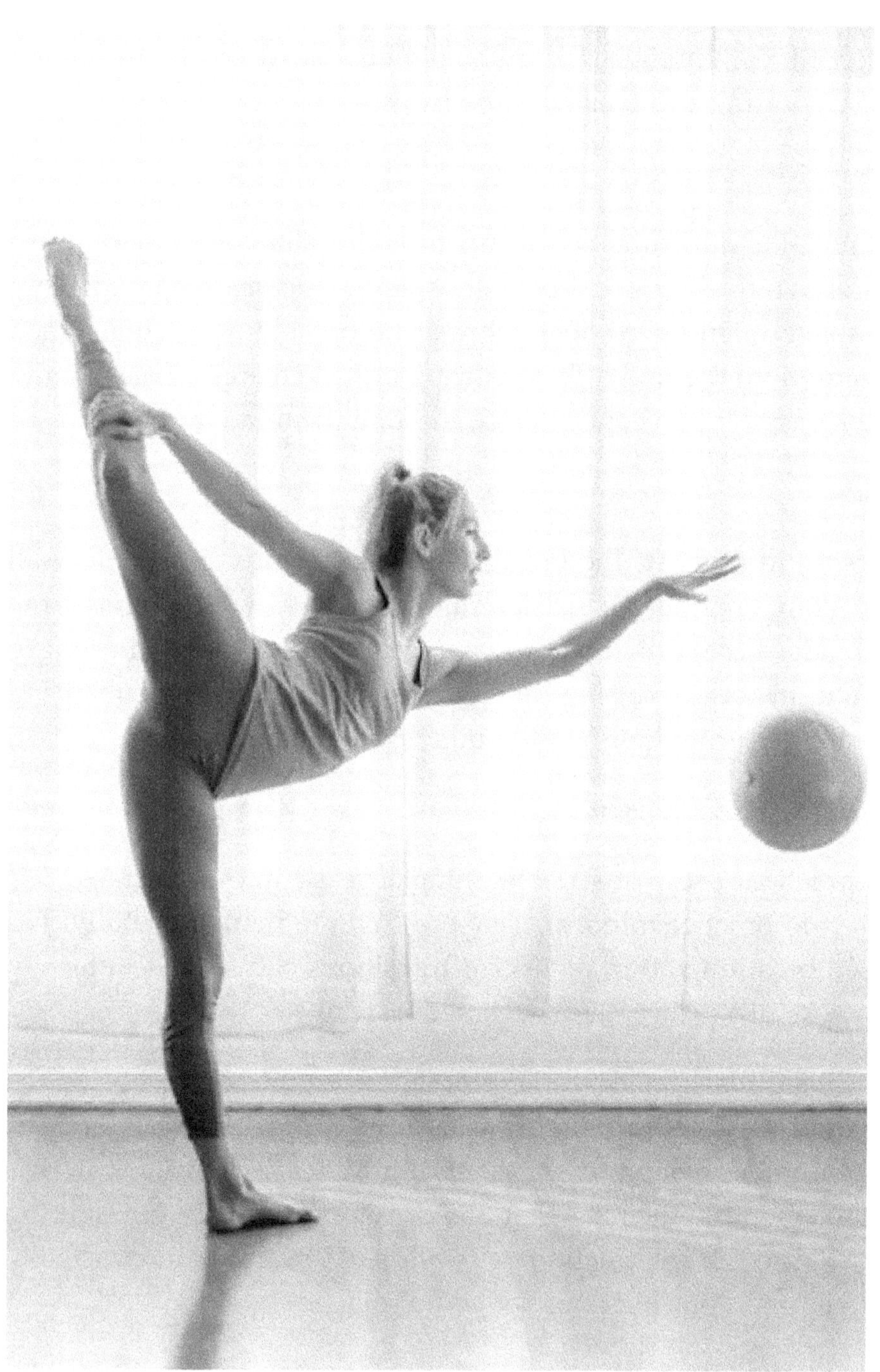

1. Starting a Self-Discovery Journey:

Determining your body's boundaries requires a deep, reflective trip. With a unique combination of strength, flexibility, and mobility, each person sets out on a personal Wall Pilates journey. This voyage is an invitation to explore your body's subtleties, recognize its capabilities, acknowledge its limits, and embrace the changing terrain of your physicality.

2. Practicing Mindfulness on the Mat:

Practicing mindfulness is The key to becoming aware of your body's limitations on the mat. Turn your focus inside when doing Wall Pilates routines. Pay attention to your body's subtle signs, such as sensations, feelings of comfort or pain, and changes in your energy levels. This awareness of yourself is the map that leads you across the terrain of your own body, enabling you to move through it purposefully and sensitively.

3. Aware of Individual Comfort Zones:

Wall Pilates promotes discovery and development with various exercises. But even in this vast landscape, there are places where you may feel safe and in alignment with your body—personal comfort zones. Understanding and honoring these zones is essential. It recognizes the value of laying a foundation before pursuing new endeavors rather than advocating stagnation. These comfort zones are where a strong foundation for advancement is established.

4. Differing Between Pain and Discomfiture:

Determining between discomfort and agony is essential to knowing your body's limitations. Pain, often a necessary component of challenging workouts, indicates that your muscles are working and changing. Contrarily, pain is an alert system that should never be disregarded. You may safely push limits and avoid being hurt by distinguishing between the two. When an activity causes discomfort, it's a signal to change, amend, or stop doing that specific action.

5. Valuing Personal Flexibility and Mobility:

Wall Pilates recognizes that each practitioner's range of mobility and flexibility is unique and embraces this uniqueness. Respecting your range of motion entails being aware of your body's limitations. Focus on your body's journey rather than imitate someone else's stretch or stance. As your body changes, work within the confines of your existing mobility, progressively increasing it. By treating your body with respect, you may develop a healthy connection with its natural powers.

6. Identifying Your Advantages and Disadvantages:

Knowing your body's limitations is more than just being aware of its physical limitations; it also entails knowing your advantages and disadvantages. Honor the parts of your body that work well, such as your balance, flexibility, or core strength. Address areas that can be more difficult at the same time. This balanced awareness promotes general improvement by enabling a focused and comprehensive approach to your Wall Pilates practice.

7. Assisting with Intensity Modification Based on Energy Levels:

The body is a dynamic being impacted by more than just its physical makeup. Realizing your body's limitations means accepting that your energy levels will fluctuate. Your body can want higher intensity on certain days and milder action on others. Based on your energy levels, modify the intensity of your Wall Pilates exercise to create a harmonious and long-lasting connection with your body.

8. Appreciating Advancement with Patience:

P og R session in the Wall Pilates is a process rather than a final goal. It's a careful balance between accepting patience and pushing limits. Understand that the body changes at a unique rate. As you practice regularly, acknowledge and appreciate your minor achievements. Fostering a feeling of success without giving in to the pressure of quick development is the key to mastering the skill of knowing your body's limitations.

9. Developing Positive Body Language:

Our experience and perception of our bodies are shaped by how we describe them. Being aware of your body's limitations requires you to develop body-positive language. Affirmations that acknowledge the work and resiliency that are intrinsic to your practice should take the place of self-criticism. This mental adjustment fosters a supportive atmosphere that advances rather than impedes your path of self-discovery and development.

10. Looking for Professional Assistance and Guidance:

Starting to realize your body's limitations is made more accessible by getting help from a specialist. As with any exercise regimen, getting advice from a certified teacher or medical expert regarding Wall Pilates may be very insightful. Their knowledge helps you customize your practice to meet your requirements and ensure you are guided by expertise while you explore the boundaries of your body.

11. Switching to New Circumstances:

Like life, the body is prone to change. Being flexible in the face of shifting conditions is essential to knowing your body's limitations. A change in your health, an injury, or an incident in life might affect your practice. Instead of fighting change, modify your Wall Pilates routine as necessary. Exercise modifications, intensity adjustments, and a flexible mentality that respects the constantly changing nature of your physical body are all important aspects of practicing yoga.

12. Promoting a Holistic Perspective:

In the end, realizing your body's limitations in Wall Pilates is an all-encompassing practice that goes beyond the gym. It also entails caring for the mind, soul, and body. Develop a healthy connection with your body, become more self-aware, and accept the interconnectedness of holistic well-being. As you set out on this path, realize that being aware of your body's limitations is a continuous process of inquiry—a graceful dance of self-awareness, development, and constant self-compassion.

Knowing your body's limitations becomes a story in the lyrical language of Wall Pilates—a tale of thoughtful investigation, resiliency, and the changing fabric of your well-being. It is evidence of the knowledge that arises from a harmonic conversation between the body and the intellect, which creates a haven where the boundaries of the present become the opportunities of the future.

Chapter 2: Core Strengthening Basics

2.1: Wall Roll-Down

A classic Pilates exercise, the Wall Roll-Down is a symphony of deliberate movement, spine articulation, and conscious breathing. The Wall Roll-Down is a cornerstone exercise in the fascinating world of Wall Pilates. It's a graceful way to start a session focusing on strength, flexibility, and body-mind awareness. Together, we will delve into the subtleties of the Wall Roll-Down and examine how these details turn this exercise into a creative way to represent Pilates philosophy.

1. Starting the Motion:

With an elegant beginning that features standing tall against the wall, the Wall Roll-Down gets underway. To create a solid base, ground yourself by standing with your feet hip-width apart and contracting your core. Imagine your spine lengthening as you take a deep breath and see the top of your head reaching toward the ceiling. This first stage is a preparation breath that gives the body energy and attentiveness.

2. Spine Articulation:

The precise articulation of the spine, which unfolds with intentional precision, is the characteristic of the Wall Roll-Down. Breathe slowly, letting your chin drop to your chest to begin moving from the topmost vertebrae in your spine. Imagine a cascading effect when each vertebra separates from the wall, resulting in a smooth and graceful drop. The exercise demonstrates how the Pilates concept of spinal mobility promotes control and flexibility.

3. Preserving Fundamental Engagement:

A continuous companion throughout the Wall Roll-Down is core engagement. The movement is stabilized by the deep contraction of the abdominal muscles, especially the transverse abdominis, which also forms a corset that supports the spine. This core engagement enables a regulated, segmental spine movement and prevents collapse during the controlled descent.

4. Forging a Flexible Bond:

The Wall Roll-Down is a dance, a fluid fusion of movement and breath. The exhalation directs the descent by providing a continuous thread that passes through the articulations of each vertebra. How the movement flows and reflects the breath creates a rhythmic flow that transforms the exercise into a moving meditation. This flowing relationship promotes a deep feeling of awareness in addition to physical coordination.

5. Observing the Alignment:

Alignment in the Wall Roll-Down is visual poetry. Note how each vertebra aligns with the wall when the spine articulates. The objective is to keep the trajectory on course without experiencing any sudden changes or misalignments. You may fine-tune the movement and develop a more acute awareness of the spine's trip with the help of the wall's visual feedback.

6. Delighting in the Progression Fold

A forward fold marks the peak of the fall, a sign of release and surrender. Keep your knees slightly bent while your body gently folds forward to avoid putting too much strain on your lower back. The invitation to enjoy the stretch throughout the hamstrings, the spine, and the whole posterior chain comes with the forward fold. Accept the feeling of your body opening up and stretching through the back.

7. Understanding the Extension:

Investigate the stretch for a little while as your body hangs elegantly in the front fold. Sensate the back gently opening, the shoulders becoming less tense, and the spine lengthening. In this phase, the Wall Roll-Down transforms into a meditative pause, a time to slow down, breathe deeply, let go of any remaining tension, and enjoy the sensation of spaciousness produced inside the body.

8. Ordering by Sequence:

In the Wall Roll-Down, the climb is a purposeful reversal of the drop, executed sequentially. To start, tighten your core and let your vertebrae stack on each other, slowly rolling back up the wall. Sequential unwinding provides a smooth and balanced return to the upright posture by mirroring the previous articulation in reverse.

9. Conscious Reestablishing:

Enjoy the attentive reconnection with an upright posture as you stand tall against the wall once again. Beyond its obvious physical advantages, the Wall Roll-Down transforms into a symbolic experience — a cyclical investigation of climb and down that reflects the cycles of life. The exercise's intentionality — a deliberate return to the present moment with an awakened awareness of the body and breath — is highlighted by this attentive reconnection.

10. Accessibility Modifications for R:

Although the Wall Roll-Down is elegant and demanding, it may be modified to suit varying fitness levels or physical limitations. Regular practice may adjust the descent to a comfortable range for those with restricted flexibility. Adding props to your exercises, such as a little Pilates ball between your thighs, will boost your interest and provide more support.

11. Including in the Pilates Exercise:

The Wall Roll-Down is a fundamental exercise included in a Pilates practice rather than being practiced alone. It works well as a dynamic stretch as well as a warm-up for a variety of activities. Its focus on core engagement, rhythmic flow, and spinal articulation provides the foundation for later exercises, resulting in a cohesive and well-rounded Pilates session.

12. Building the Mind-Body Bond:

Beyond its health advantages, the Wall Roll-Down is a perfect example of Pilates' core practice—a profound development of the mind-body connection. Every movement, breath, and vertebral articulation invites one to become more aware of the present moment and the limits and potential of one's own body. With its gracefulness, the Wall Roll-Down opens the door to the transforming possibilities that arise when movement and awareness are combined.

The Wall Roll-Down's exquisite choreography uses the body as a canvas and the movement as a brushstroke to create a story of embodied awareness, power, and flexibility. With its beautiful simplicity, this fundamental exercise embodies the Pilates philosophy, which goes beyond the workout and develops into a thoughtful journey of complete well-being.

2.2: Standing Leg Lifts

Standing leg lifts are a powerful and elegant exercise in the Wall Pilates repertoire that demonstrates balance, strength, and accuracy. These leg lifts become a pillar of Pilates choreography, combining the difficulty of unilateral leg movement with the wall's grounding support. In this article, we will examine the subtleties of Standing Leg Lifts and how they may be used to sculpt the lower body and demonstrate attentive movement.

1. Postural Alignment's Basis:

The first step in doing Standing Leg Lifts is to build a solid foundation. This alignment is similar to the Pilates notion of having an extended spine and a sturdy core. Make sure your feet are hip-width apart as you stand tall and lean on the wall. As you move your navel softly toward your spine with your engaged core muscles, release your shoulders and allow your spine to retain its curvature naturally. This basic alignment prepares the body for the graceful leg lifts that come next.

2. Core Activation Done Gently:

In Pilates, the core is the center of strength, and standing leg lifts target this powerhouse effectively. Keep your core muscles lightly activated as you prepare for the leg lifts. This delicate interaction helps maintain the spine, which permits deliberate motion and prevents the lower back from rounding or arching. The subtle stimulation of the core is the anchor for the graceful leg lifts.

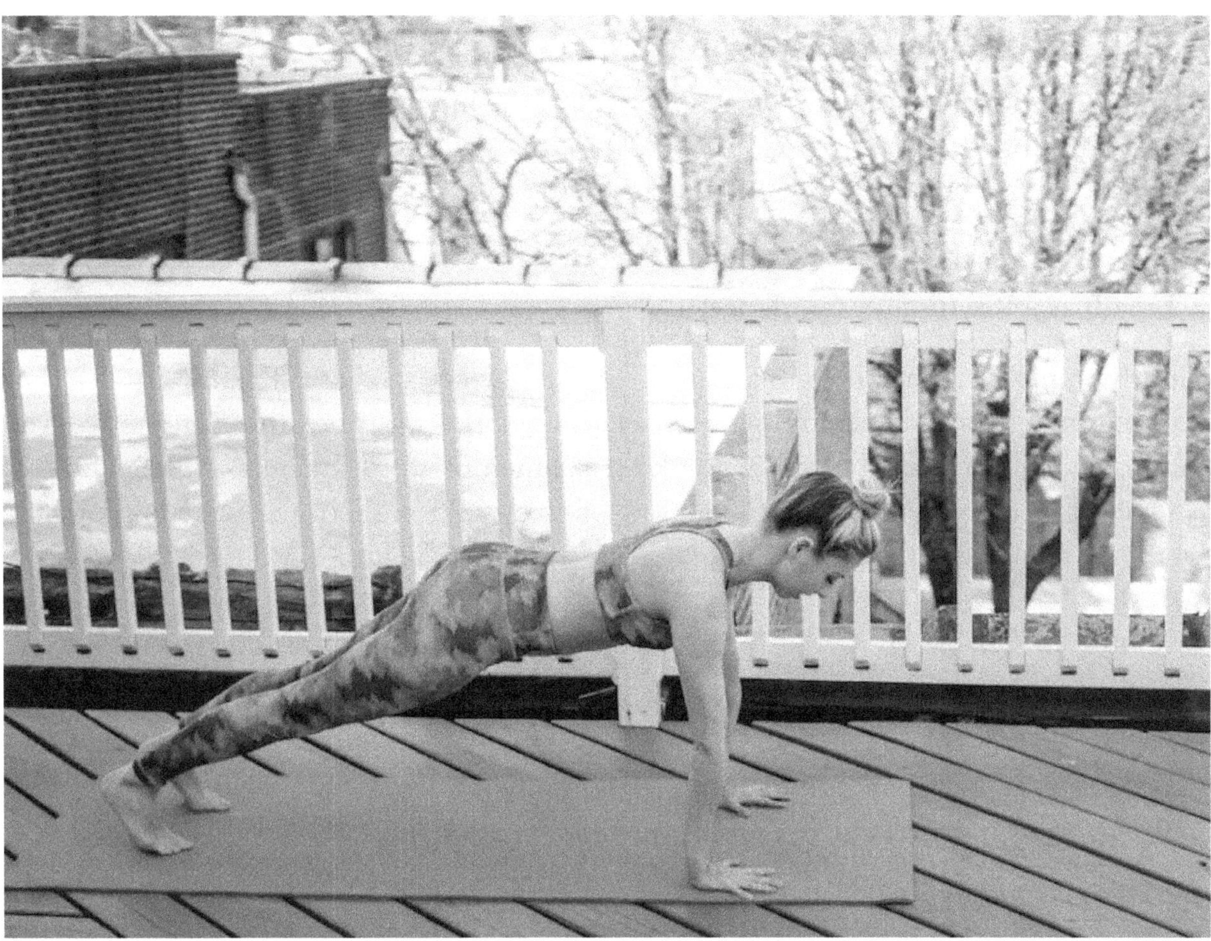

3. Squatting Against the Wall:

Try slanting a little toward the wall to improve stability and provide more support. This modification aids in balance maintenance and frees up your mind to concentrate on the deliberate engagement of the standing leg. The wall becomes a reliable ally, providing a point of contact that promotes alignment and balance and guarantees a smooth performance of the leg lifts.

4. Leg Lifts with Contours:

The working leg's intentional and controlled movement makes Standing Leg Lifts effective. Lift the leg to hip height or higher, starting at the hip and keeping the knee straight. The hip flexors and quadriceps must contract for the action to have purpose and avoid momentum. Not only do the regulated leg lifts tone the lower body, but they also increase body awareness.

5. Keeping the Pelvis Neutral:

Stress keeps the pelvis neutral as the working leg rises. Steer clear of excessive pelvic tilting or rotation, and ensure the action starts at the hip joint. In addition to supporting the hip flexors' focused activation, the neutral pelvis promotes the lower body's harmonic engagement. This alignment concept is consistent with Pilates's balanced and controlled movement cornerstone.

6. Breath as a Rhythm for Guidance:

The rhythmic element of the Standing Leg Lift dance is breath. Breathe in to prime yourself, then release as you raise the leg. This will bring your breathing and movement into harmony. The breath gives the workout a contemplative element and aids with core activation. A smooth and continuous flow of energy throughout the body is promoted by the deliberate exhale, which stimulates the muscles to contract and rise.

7. Pay Attention to Hip Abduction:

Standing leg lifts primarily focus on hip abduction or the leg's outward motion away from the body's midline. This concentration activates the gluteus medius and other outside hip muscles. Not only do these muscles help to contour the hips, but they also improve stability and promote the best possible function throughout everyday tasks.

8. Conscientious Leg Lowering:

The deliberate lowering of the leg is just as significant as the lift. Avoid giving in to the urge to let the leg fall suddenly. Instead, descend the leg deliberately, stressing the activation of the hip flexors and preserving the pelvic position. The whole-body aspect of Standing Leg Lifts is completed by the eccentric part of the action during the descent, which enhances muscular strength and control.

9. Examination of Different

Standing Leg Lifts provide space for experimentation and advancement. After mastering the essential exercise, consider varying it to work with other lower body parts. This can include experimenting with various angles, adding ankle weights for resistance, or investigating dynamic variants that include deliberate pulsating motions. Exercise depth is increased by variations, which guarantee a steady improvement in strength and flexibility.

10. Equilibrium Bilateral Cooperation:

Standing Leg Lifts emphasize the working leg above all else, but the supporting leg must also be balanced naturally. To maintain balance and alignment, the standing leg serves as a stabilizer, using the quadriceps, core, and inner thigh muscles. This bilateral involvement enhances general lower body strength and stability while guaranteeing a symmetrical exercise.

11. The Integration of Mindful Awareness:

Standing Leg Lifts take on depth and meaning when done with mindful awareness. Focus on the feelings in the working thigh and hip as you raise and drop the leg. Take note of the breath, the deliberate movement, and the use of muscles. Exercise becomes a thoughtful journey instead of just a physical activity when mindful awareness is applied, strengthening the connection between the body and the mind.

12. Combining into a Whole Pilates Program:

Standing Leg Lifts are a foundational exercise for a full-body lower-body workout that easily fits into any Pilates program. They may be mixed and matched with other exercises focusing on various muscle groups to create a Pilates session that works in unison. This integration guarantees a comprehensive exercise program that targets balance, strength, and flexibility throughout the body.

Standing leg lifts provide the following advantages:

1. **Hip Stability and Strength:** By focusing on the hip muscles, standing leg lifts help to strengthen and stabilize the hip joint.
2. **Core Activation:** By working the core muscles, the exercise improves stability and strength throughout the body.

3. **Muscle growth:** The lower body's muscular growth is balanced due to the active involvement of the working and supporting legs.
4. **Enhanced Body Awareness:** The deliberate technique and movement foster an elevated body awareness, encouraging a stronger connection between the body and mind.
5. **Improved Hip Flexibility:** The dynamic leg lifts increase hip flexibility, which helps with everyday tasks by enhancing the range of motion.

Standing Leg Lifts are a beautiful expression of power, balance, and conscious movement in the elegant language of Wall Pilates. It transforms from a workout into a journey as the leg rises gently against the wall's support. This journey sculpts the lower body, cultivates attentive awareness, and reveals the elegance of Pilates in each deliberate movement.

2.3: Wall Planks

A staple of the Pilates repertoire, wall planks are a dynamic combination of strength, stability, and awareness. Wall Planks, rooted in Pilates concepts, use the wall's support to provide a controlled intensity and full-body activation platform. Let's dissect this workout and examine the minute elements that turn Wall Planks into a shaping symphony for the shoulders, core, and general stability.

1. Initial Alignment and Posture:

Starting with Wall Planks needs alignment and a grounded stance. Assume a facing position with your feet hip-width apart. With your palms firmly pushing against the wall, place your hands at shoulder height against it. Reposition your feet while keeping your head and heels in alignment until your body forms a straight line. This warm-up position creates a solid base prepared for the challenge of the following plank position.

2. Activation of the Core Muscles:

Engaging the core muscles is what makes Wall Planks unique. Use your abdominal muscles, especially the transverse abdominis, while you press up against the wall in a plank posture. This engagement helps to maintain a continuous line from the head to the heels and prevents drooping in the lower back by providing a sturdy foundation for the plank. The exercise's overall tone is established by activating the core, which is the anchor.

3. Stability and Alignment of the Shoulders:

In wall planks, shoulder alignment is crucial. Ensure your wrists and shoulders are precisely above each other to form a vertical support line. Shoulder girdle engagement, which involves the upper back muscles, stabilizes the shoulders and reduces needless strain. This position improves shoulder stability and strength while maximizing the exercise's efficacy.

4. Pelvic Alignment and Neutral Spine:

One of the main ideas of wall planks is to maintain a neutral spine. Steer clear of severe back curvature or arching, and keep a straight spine. Concurrently, be mindful of your pelvic position. The pelvis should neither be drooping downward nor tilted upward about the spine. Precise attention to the alignment of the spine and pelvis guarantees the best possible activation of the core muscles and facilitates a secure and efficient plank posture.

5. Linear Advancement to Complete Plank:

It's advised to take things slowly if you're new to Wall Planks or want to make changes. Start with a modified plank to give your body time to adjust to the effort needed for the exercise. Work your way up to a complete plank posture as your strength and stability grow. By taking little steps, you can guarantee that your body adapts to the demands of the activity without being overexercised.

6. Inhaling with a Coordinated Cadence:

In Wall Planks, breathing becomes a coordinated rhythm that synchronizes with the demands of the workout. Breathe deeply through your nose to expand your rib cage. Then, release your breath through pursed lips to contract your core muscles. In addition to improving oxygenation, this regular breathing pattern keeps the plank stable. With the breath acting as a steady anchor, the dynamic intensity of the exercise takes on a contemplative element.

7. Equal Foot Position and Weight Distribution:

In wall planks, the distribution of weight is crucial. Ensure your weight is split equally between your hands and shoulders to prevent putting too much strain on your wrists. Remember to consider your foot placement. Having the feet hip-width apart provides the ideal alignment and a secure basis. An intentional distribution of weight and placement of the feet help create a regulated and balanced plank stance.

8. Extending the Spine:

In Wall Planks, elongation of the spine is a modest but essential feature. Feel your spine extend as you imagine the top of your head reaching toward the wall. This elongation promotes a conscious awareness of the body's alignment and increases the exercise's efficacy. The spine turns into a support system for stability and strength.

9. Adjustments for Various Intensities:

Wall Planks provide a range of intensities. To make it more difficult, think of raising your feet to create an angled plank stance on a step or platform. This adjustment increases the upper body, shoulders, and core involvement. Conversely, the plank may be done with the hands higher on the wall to lessen effort or accommodate constraints. These adaptations provide accessibility and progression for a range of fitness levels.

10. Stillness and Moderated Dissension:

Gaining endurance with Wall Planks is a logical next step. Focus on keeping your shoulders stable and your core engaged as you hold the plank posture. Gradually, endurance builds with regular practice. Avoid letting go or falling while finishing the plank. Instead, descend mindfully while highlighting the activation of your core and the deliberate lowering of your body. This deliberate division elegantly closes the task.

Advantages of Wall Planks:

1. **Core Strength:** Wall Planks work the whole abdominal area, making them an excellent tool for developing core strength.
2. **Shoulder Stability:** This exercise develops strength and stability by focusing on the upper back and shoulder muscles.
3. **Total Body Engagement:** Wall planks provide a thorough full-body exercise by engaging the arms, legs, and back, among other muscle groups.
4. **Spinal Alignment:** Postural awareness is encouraged by emphasizing a neutral spine and improving spinal alignment.
5. **Adaptability:** Wall Planks may be modified to meet various people's demands and fitness levels.
6. **Mind-Body Connection:** Wall Planks practiced mindfully, which leads to a deeper awareness of breath, body alignment, and general presence.

Wall Planks become a composition, a symphony of strength, stability, and focused participation in the elegant language of Pilates. The body becomes a monument to the complex interaction between the physical and the conscious as it shapes into a robust plank against the wall's support. Wall Planks are a tool for body sculpting. Still, they also tell a story of resiliency, accuracy, and the lasting power that results from the union of the mind and body in deliberate movement.

2.4: Pelvic Tilts

A staple of the Wall Pilates repertory, pelvic tilts are a transformational exercise that explores the subtleties of lumbar stability and core engagement. Pelvic tilts are:

- A bridge in the elegant language of Pilates.
- We are connecting movements.
- Breath.
- The complex dance of the pelvis.

Join us as we explore the intricacies that make Pelvic Tilts an essential exercise for building a solid core and supporting lumbar health. Join us as we travel through the art and benefits of this exercise.

1. Posture and Grounding at First:

The Pelvic tilt journey begins with a deliberate anchoring of the body. As you stand with your back to the wall, gently activate your core and keep your spine neutral. A sturdy base is created by placing the feet hip-width apart. This first position aligns with the wall's support and invites a conscious presence to start the next pelvic movement.

2. Starting the Slope:

The intentional tilting of the pelvis is the core of Pelvic Tilts. Take a deep breath and let the breath initiate the tilt. Tilt your pelvis slightly as you release the breath, pressing your lower back into the wall. To do this action, the transverse abdominis and other abdominal muscles must be slightly engaged, and the pelvis must be articulated carefully. The slow beginning gives the pelvic tilt a feeling of elegance and flow.

3. Sequential Spinal Movement:

Pelvic tilts are a series of movements that start at the pelvis and work their way up the spine. Imagine the lumbar spine progressively sinking as the pelvis tilts backwards, then the thoracic spine. There is no change in the cervical spine's neutral position. This exercise is more fluid overall because the action is performed sequentially, guaranteeing a harmonic spine articulation.

4. Activation of the Core Muscles:

To intensify the action, contract your core muscles at the peak of the pelvic tilt. The internal obliques, transverse abdominis, and pelvic floor muscles form a corset of support that encircles the pelvis. This interaction helps shape the abdominal area and makes the tilt more intense. The Pilates concept of centring is embodied by the core, which becomes a stabilizing force.

5. Extending the Spine:

Focus on the extension of the spine at the same time as engaging the core. Imagine the top of the head stretching toward the ceiling while the pelvis tilts back, extending the whole spine. This lengthening is an important detail that encourages the body to feel roomy and aligned. The spine turns into a channel for elegance and power.

6. Conscientious Range Exploration:

Pelvic tilts encourage a deliberate investigation of the pelvic region's range of motion. Though tilting the pelvis backwards is the main action, pay attention to your body's specific range of motion and comfort level. The intention is to foster a delicate inquiry that respects the limits of the body rather than to push the movement. This awareness-based method cultivates a stronger connection with the body's intelligence.

7. An Equitable Hip Engagement:

Pelvic tilt movement is radiated by the hips, including the anterior and posterior regions. The glutes contract, and the hip flexors extend as the pelvis tilts rearward. Targeting the flexors and extensors of the hips, this balanced hip engagement guarantees a comprehensive exercise. Reciprocity between these muscle groups supports the lumbar region and helps maintain pelvic stability.

8. Managed Reversion to Neutral:

The pelvic Tilt trip is complete with a deliberate return to neutral. Breathe deeply in, then slowly relax the pelvic tilt as you exhale, allowing the spine to naturally level itself against the wall. The deliberate return highlights the intentional quality of the movement and offers a chance to see the minute changes in the body.

9. Breath in Pelvic Tilts:

Breath acts as a guiding rhythm, coordinating with the action. Breathe in to get ready and out as you begin the pelvic tilt. The exhale encourages a sensation of release and surrender into the action and facilitates core engagement. The dynamic simplicity of Pelvic Tilts takes on a contemplative dimension as the breath becomes a friend.

10. Variations in Intensity:

Pelvic tilts are versatile, allowing adjustments to suit varying degrees of fitness. Consider adding a little lift of the feet off the ground during the pelvic tilt for individuals looking for more intensity. This change defies equilibrium and increases the core's participation. On the other hand, those who prefer a more delicate method may execute the exercise with a reduced range of motion, progressively increasing it via regular repetition.

Pelvic tilt benefits:

1. **Activation of the Core:** Pelvic tilts aggressively activate the core muscles, enhancing stability and strength.
2. **Lumbar Support:** Deliberate movement helps to create a supporting environment for the lower back by promoting lumbar stability.
3. **Spinal Articulation:** The spine's progressive motion improves spinal articulation, which fosters alignment and flexibility.
4. **Balanced Hip Engagement:** Pelvic tilts provide a flat hip engagement by working the hip flexors and extensors.
5. **Attentive Body Connection:** Pelvic tilts' purposeful, focused design fosters a more acute awareness of the alignment and movement of the body.
6. **Accessible for All Levels:** Due to its versatility, Pelvic Tilts may be customized to meet the demands of persons with various fitness levels.

Pelvic tilts become a lyrical movement in the elegant Pilates choreography, a ballet between breath, core activation, and spinal articulation. The pelvis becomes a canvas on which stability and strength are purposefully painted when it tilts backwards toward the wall. In their simplicity, pelvic tilts reveal the deep connection between movement, breath, and the creative quality of the moving body.

2.5: Wall Sit with Abdominal Engagement

An exercise that combines lower body endurance and core activation is the Wall Sit with Abdominal Engagement, which embodies the synergy found in Wall Pilates. It is an engaging workout. In the elegant language of Pilates, this exercise blends the dynamic engagement of the abdominal muscles with the isometric strain of a wall sit. Now, let's explore the subtleties of the Wall Sit with Abdominal Engagement and how strength, stability, and core power create a beautiful movement.

1. Readiness and Wall Sitting Position:

A basic Wall Sit posture is needed to begin the Wall Sit with Abdominal Engagement. Make sure your feet are hip-width apart as you stand with your back to the wall. Lower your torso and bend your knees as you slide down the wall until your thighs parallel the floor. Here, the focus is on producing a straight line with the hips, knees, and ankles and a right angle at the knees. This warm-up posture creates the foundation for the wall's isometric difficulty.

2. Initiation of Abdominal Engagement:

Concentrate on the beginning of the abdominal contraction as you get comfortable in the Wall Sit. To get ready, take a deep breath, then slowly move your navel toward your spine as you exhale. By purposefully engaging the abdominal muscles, the standard wall sit becomes a more comprehensive exercise that uses the core as a stabilizing mechanism. Core strength and lower body endurance are connected when the abs are contracted.

3. Building a Support Corset:

The Wall Sit's abdominal engagement acts as the body's corset of support. The pelvic floor muscles, internal obliques, and transverse abdominis provide a solid base. This activation, which resembles a corset, increases wall sit endurance and ensures the lower back is supported, avoiding undue strain or arching. Strength and restrained power interact dynamically during the Wall Sit with Abdominal Engagement.

4. Keeping the Alignment:

When doing the Wall Sit with Abdominal Engagement, alignment is crucial. Ensure your whole spine is supported and your back is flush with the wall. The goal is to keep the spine neutral and free of any rounding or arching. The thighs should parallel the floor, and the knees should be just above the ankles. This meticulous attention to alignment maximizes the efficiency of the wall sit and abdominal engagement.

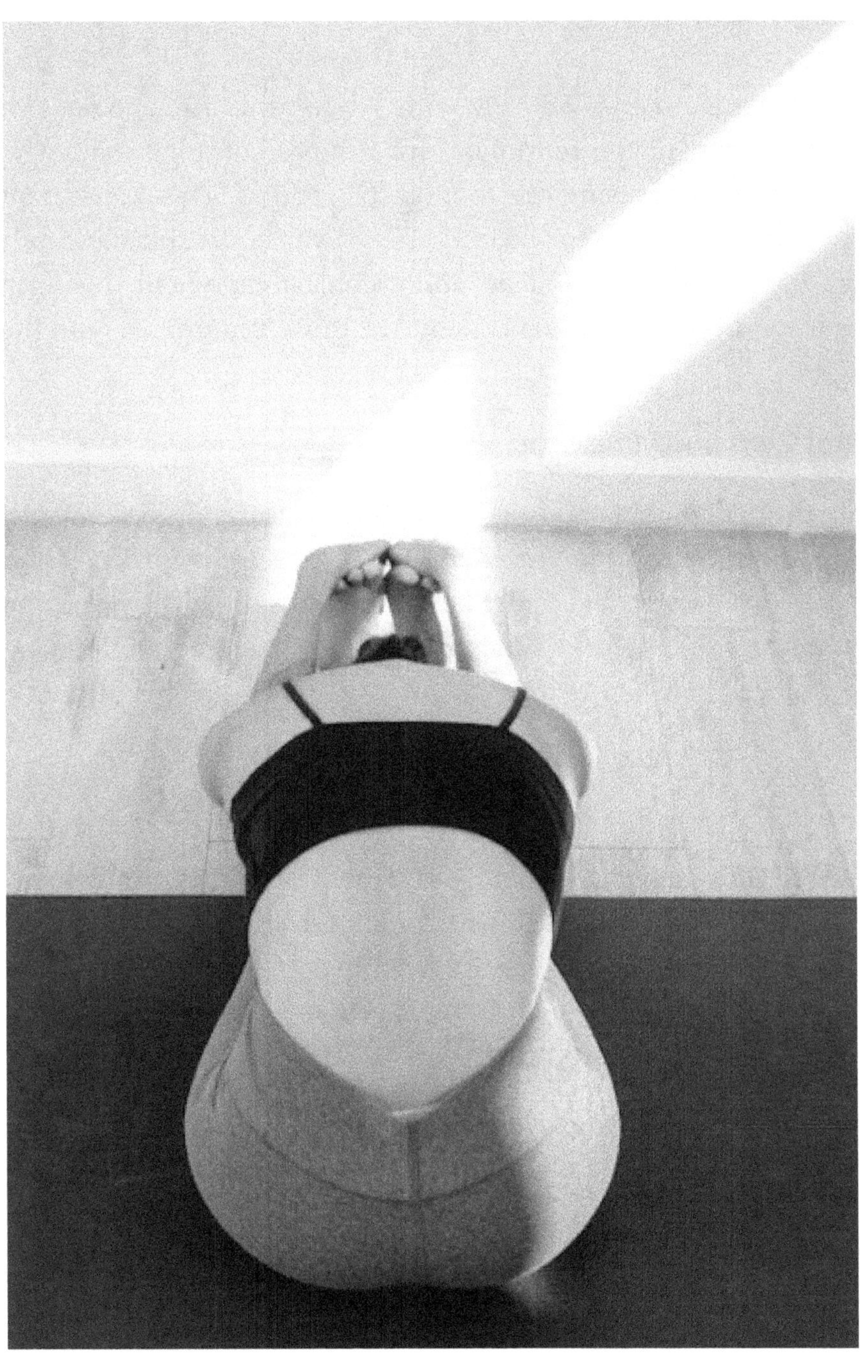

5. Breath as a Harmonious Foundation:

In the Wall Sit with Abdominal Engagement, the breath plays a crucial function as a rhythmic anchor throughout the exercise. Please take a deep breath to be ready, then release it as you contract your abdominal muscles. The wall sit's endurance is increased by the rhythmic exhalation, which also helps to activate the core. In the isometric challenge, the breath takes on a meditative rhythm that promotes ease and control.

6. Intensity Variations:

Changes in intensity may be made to the Wall Sit with Abdominal Engagement to accommodate different fitness levels. If you're looking for a more complex challenge, try keeping your wall sit position while raising one foot off the ground. This adjustment adds a degree of instability, increasing the workload on the lower body and the core's involvement. On the other hand, concentrating on abdominal engagement during a conventional wall sit offers a solid basis for advancement for those unfamiliar with the activity.

7. Long-Term Durability and Conscious Presence:

The Wall Sit with Abdominal Engagement requires mental presence and goes beyond just physical endurance. Pay attention to how your abdominal muscles contract as you maintain the wall sit. Sensual stimulation, a supportive corset around the belly, and the growth of lower body endurance are all felt. The exercise becomes an integrated feeling of strength and awareness rather than just a mechanical wall sit when this attentive presence is present.

8. Elegant Fall and Rise:

Transition gracefully to the Wall Sit with Abdominal Engagement's conclusion. To stand up straight, take a deep breath, relax your abs, and push through your legs. The recovery phase emphasizes regulated movement and a smooth transition to a standing posture. It is a graceful drop from the isometric challenge. This deliberate recuperation enhances the exercise's strength-building component.

Advantages of Wall Sitting with Engaged Abs:

1. **Lower Body Endurance:** By concentrating on the quadriceps, hamstrings, and glutes, the wall sit component works the lower body endurance.
2. **Core Activation:** Abdominal engagement provides a dynamic element by engaging the transverse abdominis, internal obliques, and pelvic floor muscles.
3. **Stabilization of the Lower Back:** By creating corset-like support via abdominal engagement, the lower back is stabilized, and pain or strain is avoided.
4. **Improved Posture:** Better posture results from both abdominal engagement and the wall sit's emphasis on alignment.
5. **Mind-Body Connection:** By engaging the lower body and core synchronistically, one may cultivate awareness and presence via a deeper mind-body connection.
6. **Versatility for All Fitness Levels:** The workout is scalable and accessible because of its versatility, which enables adaptations to suit all fitness levels.

The Wall Sit with Abdominal Engagement becomes a duet, a complex dance between lower body strength and core power, in the graceful choreography of Wall Pilates. The deliberate activation of the abdominals as the body descends into the wall sit transforms the exercise from a static stance to a dynamic synthesis of controlled engagement and endurance. The Wall Sit with Abdominal Engagement shows the seamless fusion of elegance and power within the Pilates paradigm.

2.6: Side Plank with Wall Support

A dynamic combination of lateral strength and core stability, the Side Plank with Wall Support is a beautiful jewel in the Wall Pilates tapestry. This exercise delivers a unique combination of isometric challenge and conscious participation because of its strong origins in Pilates concepts. Let's examine the nuances of the Side Plank with Wall Support, revealing the layers that contribute to its foundational role in shaping the lateral core and promoting a balanced body.

1. Initial Wall Support and Positioning:

Starting the Side Plank with Wall Support requires careful placement. Laying on your side, position your hips, shoulders, and feet on the wall to start. The wall gives the body a solid base of support, laying the groundwork for the next lateral challenge. The lower arm and shoulder should be at a straight angle, with the lower arm being perpendicular to the torso. This initial posture prepares The body for the side plank's dynamic strength and stability.

2. Activation of the Core Muscles:

The activation of the core muscles starts the trip toward the Side Plank with Wall Support. To engage the transverse abdominis and internal obliques, bring your navel slightly toward your spine as you raise your hips off the floor. The exercise's fundamental focus is this core activation, stabilizing the body. The wall's support is a guiding anchor, enabling deliberate activation of the lateral core muscles and controlled movement.

3. Creating a Straight Line and Lifting the Hips:

Raising the hips is an essential part of the Side plan with Wall Support. Keep your head and heels straight as you raise your hips. The obliques and quadratus lumborum cooperate to engage the lateral portion of the body. The wall's support is a reminder to stay aligned and avoid drooping or deviating from the straight line. With this deliberate lift, the exercise becomes a dynamic demonstration of lateral strength.

4. Stability and Alignment of the Shoulders:

In the Side Plank with Wall Support, shoulder alignment is crucial. Ensure the arm you use for support—the one on the ground—is positioned exactly behind your shoulder. By aligning the shoulder joint, excessive strain is avoided, and stability is maximized. The upper back and shoulder girdle muscles work together to sustain the body's weight actively. The wall provides stability, which makes it possible to execute the side plank with assurance and control.

5. Neck Alignment and Gaze:

Lift your head and keep your neck in a neutral position. The head should not tilt or rotate excessively; instead, it should be in alignment with the spine. Maintaining a regulated alignment of the neck helps preserve the integrity of the spine by avoiding needless pressure on the cervical spine. During the practice, the gaze becomes a focused point, improving awareness and concentration.

6. Breath as a Calm Respite:

Breath takes on a supporting cadence in the Side Plank with Wall Support dynamic hold. Breathe deeply to be ready, then release as you raise your hips and use your core. Breathing rhythmically helps to both activate the abdominal muscles and provide a feeling of comfort in the face of difficulty. Breath becomes a guiding rhythm, allowing breath and movement to harmonize.

7. Differences for the Progressive Task:

There is an opportunity for advancement and challenge with the Side Plank with Wall Support. For those looking for a more challenging version, think about pulling the top leg off the bottom leg to provide even more instability. This variant throws balance and coordination off balance and escalates the lateral activity. The wall is always there to support and promote experimentation and advancement within personal fitness levels.

8. Recovering and Lowering Mindfully:

Mindfully and deliberately descend your hips as you get to the end of the Side Plank. As you return your hips to the floor, take a deep breath and slowly relax your core. The recuperation stage emphasizes the whole range of motion and is organized and intentional. In addition to bringing the exercise to a graceful conclusion, the deliberate lowering maintains the overall integrity of the movement pattern.

Downside Plank with Wall Support Advantages:

1. **Lateral Core Activation:** This exercise develops lateral core strength by focusing on the obliques and quadratus lumborum.

2. **Shoulder Stability:** The shoulder girdle supporting engagement improves shoulder stability.

3. **Spinal Alignment:** A straight back to the front helps maintain proper spinal alignment.

4. **Mind-Body Connection:** Breath, alignment, and lateral strength create a more profound mind-body connection.

5. **Progressive Challenge:** Variations support varying fitness levels and objectives by enabling advanced challenges.

6. **Stabilizing Wall Support:** The wall acts as a stabilizing element, giving assurance and control over the execution process.

7. **Balance and Coordination:** Complex variations make balance and coordination more difficult while incorporating a dynamic component into the workout.

The Side Plank with Wall Support is a solo that explores lateral strength, core stability, and conscious participation in the elegant choreography of Wall Pilates. The body lifts against the wall's support, turning into a purposefully painted painting with lines of stability and strength. A testimonial to the harmonic interaction between the body, the wall, and the attentive soul throughout the Pilates journey is the Side Plank with Wall Support.

2.7: Mountain Climber

One of Wall Pilate's most dynamic and energizing exercises, Mountain Climber pushes the envelope by combining cardiovascular effort and core involvement. Based on Pilates principles, this workout works the lower body, shoulders, and core via a rhythmic symphony of controlled motions. Now, let's explore the subtleties of the Mountain Climber and how it safely and encouragingly combines strength, endurance, and dynamic fluidity at Wall Pilates.

1. Wall Support and Initial Position:

Start the Mountain Climber by putting your hands shoulder-height against the wall in a plank stance. The wall gives the upper body a secure base, fostering an atmosphere that encourages deliberate movement. Ensure your body is straight from your head to your heels, with your wrists just under your shoulders. This initial position lays the basis for the dynamic challenge that follows.

2. First Alignment and Core Activation:

The stimulation of the core is what makes the Mountain Climber what it is. Engage the internal obliques and transverse abdominis by drawing the navel toward the spine. The controlled movement of the legs is propelled by this core engagement, which also stabilizes the plank posture. The first alignment is critical because it emphasizes a sturdy base for the following dynamic motion and a straight line from the head to the heels.

3. Knee-to-Chest Movement in Rhythm:

Start the Mountain Climber by bringing one knee in a rhythmic and controlled way toward the chest. It feels like you're sprinting in place while keeping your board against the wall. Control and accuracy are crucial to bringing the leg toward the chest without jeopardizing the plank's alignment. The workout has cardiovascular benefits by increasing heart rate due to the rhythmic quality of the action.

4. Changing Up Your Leg Movements:

The Mountain Climber is a fluid series of leg motions that alternate. As one knee returns to the beginning, quickly pull the other knee up to the chest. A smooth transition between legs is facilitated by the rhythmic alternating action, which is continuous and fluid. The regulated movement tests the body's overall balance and coordination in addition to the core.

5. Preserving Stability in the Shoulders:

Give priority to shoulder stability while doing the Mountain Climber. To avoid drooping or excessive strain, the shoulders should remain robust and stable. Activating the upper back and shoulder girdle muscles provides a stable base for dynamic leg motions. The wall acts as a stabilizing anchor, enabling a composed and confident performance.

6. Breathe in a Coordinated Pace:

The Mountain Climber's breath synchronizes to create a rhythm that complements the rapid activity. As you stay in the plank posture, please take a deep breath and release it with each knee-to-chest movement. Breathing rhythmically helps with oxygenation and improves the exercise's overall flow. The breath turns into a dependable and rhythmic partner that helps with control and endurance.

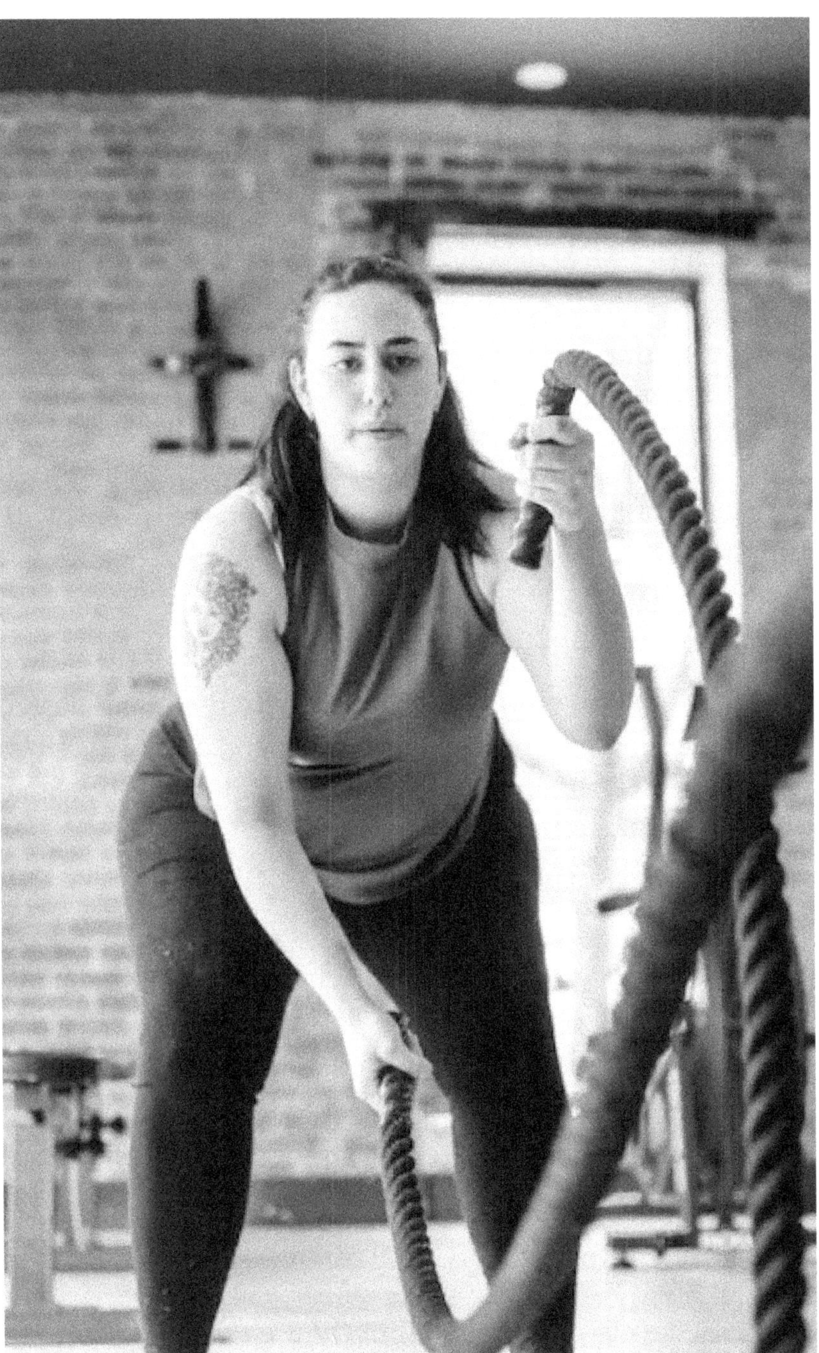

7. Mindful Presence and Regulated Pace:

Throughout the Mountain Climber, keep your pace steady and prioritize accuracy over quickness. The objectives are performing every knee-to-chest movement mindfully and maintaining the plank posture while keeping the core active. A more vital awareness of one's body's reaction to the dynamic challenge is made possible by the regulated tempo, strengthening the mind-body connection.

8. Variations in Intensity Adaptations:

Mountain Climbers may adjust to different degrees of difficulty. Try raising the feet onto a step or platform to create an angled plank stance to increase the difficulty level. This adjustment increases the shoulder and core engagement. The exercise may also be done more slowly, concentrating on controlled knee-to-chest motions for people who prefer a softer approach or to work with physical restrictions.

9. Building Endurance and Cardiovascular Effects:

The Mountain Climber's rhythmic style aids in the development of endurance. Heart rate rises with prolonged exertion, which has a cardiovascular effect. A thorough full-body exercise is produced by combining aerobic intensity and core activation with the supporting structure of Wall Pilates.

10. Humble Closure and Recuperation:

Finish the Mountain Climber by carefully lowering your knees to the floor so that you may land gracefully. Breathe deeply, letting go of the core engagement, and then return to a plank or child's pose. The exercise's deliberate finish highlights the dynamic challenge and the need for conscious healing.

Mountain Climber offers the following advantages:

1. **Core Activation:** This exercise works the whole core, which includes the rectus abdominis, transverse abdominis, and obliques.
2. **Cardiovascular Intensity:** The rhythmic leg motions raise the heart rate, which has a cardiovascular effect.
3. **Shoulder and Upper Body Engagement:** This exercise strengthens and stabilizes the upper back and shoulder girdle muscles.
4. **Coordination and Balance:** The alternating leg motions improve balance and coordination while heightening body awareness.
5. **Adaptable for Varied Fitness Levels**: Mountain climbers are flexible enough to allow for adjustments to meet a range of objectives and fitness levels.
6. **Endurance Building:** The exercises improve cardiovascular fitness by maintaining a steady beat.
7. **Entire-Body Workout:** Mountain Climbers provide an all-encompassing exercise that works the upper, lower, and core in one session.

The Mountain Climber becomes a dynamic movement in Wall Pilates' elegant choreography, a rhythmic tango between cardiovascular intensity, conscious control, and core activation. The exercise demonstrates how strength, endurance, and fluidity are seamlessly integrated within the Pilates paradigm as the legs move in rhythmic harmony against the wall's support. With the guiding principles of accuracy and mindful presence, The Mountain Climber allows practitioners to feel the rush of a full-body exercise.

Chapter 3: Lower Body Focus

3.1: Wall Squats

One of the most basic and potent exercises in the Wall Pilates repertoire, wall squats reveal the secret to building strength and stability in the lower body. This exercise, based on Pilates principles, combines the wall's supporting embrace with the dynamic challenge of a squat. Come with me as we explore the nuances of Wall Squats and how they work to build a foundation of strength by integrating controlled movement, muscle activation, and the wall's supporting force.

1. Starting the Wall Squat:

Place your back against the wall to start the Wall Squat. Ensure your feet are placed slightly away from the wall and hip-width apart. During the initiation, you will intentionally lower your body toward the ground as you descend into a squatting stance. As a guiding support, the wall permits deliberate movement while preserving alignment. This starting position creates the framework for the dynamic interaction of muscle activation throughout the squat.

2. Core Engagement and Alignment:

Pay close attention to alignment as you lower yourself into the squat. To prevent any inward collapse, the knees should track over the ankles. The wall supports the lower back gently, and the spine stays neutral. To establish a solid base, contract your core muscles simultaneously, such as the transverse abdominis and pelvic floor. Together, the alignment and core involvement provide a safe and assisted decline.

3. Forming an Angle Correctly:

Try to make a straight angle at the knees when doing the Wall Squat in an ultimately descending posture. The knees and ankles should line up, and the thighs should parallel the floor. This depth guarantees that the glutes, hamstrings, and quadriceps are well engaged. You can maximize the advantages of the squat by maintaining the correct angle, thanks to the wall's visible guidance.

4. Continuous Ascent and Decline:

The focus on deliberate movement is what makes Wall Squats so beautiful. Concentrate on using your quadriceps and glutes to enhance the action when you rise from the squat. The deliberate climb raises awareness of muscular activation while aiding in shaping the lower body muscles. The descending motion should be as intentional as the ascending motion, with the knees always positioned at the proper angle.

5. Breath as a Rhythm for Guidance:

In Wall Squats, breath acts as a guiding rhythm, coordinating with the exercise. Breathe deeply to open up your rib cage as you lower yourself into a squat. As you climb, release your breath, activating your core and pulling your navel toward your spine. The breath takes on a supporting tempo, improving the movement's fluidity and mind-body connection. The steady breathing helps you feel comfortable taking on the controlled difficulty of the squat.

6. Stability from the Wall:

The wall stabilizes during the Wall Squat, as it is always behind you. It offers a reference point for appropriate alignment, lower back support, and movement confidence. The wall's stability makes it possible for you to concentrate on using your lower body muscles without worrying about losing your balance, which makes the squat safe and efficient.

7. Targeted Areas and Muscle Engagement:

Wall squats effectively work for the lower body's major muscle groups. The main muscles that propel the climb are the quadriceps, which are found in front of the thighs. Concurrently, the hamstrings and glutes form the posterior chain by aiding in the deliberate descent and ascent. The activation of these muscles produces a toning and strengthening symphony in the lower body.

8. Variations in Intensity Adaptations:

Wall squats are versatile enough to meet various fitness levels and objectives. Try adding pulses at the bottom of the squat or holding weights at chest height to make the exercise more intense. Those who want a milder approach or have mobility issues may modify the range of motion, increasing it gradually with regular practice.

9. Intentional Movement and Mindful Presence:

Wall Squats require the practitioner to be aware of their movement's subtleties and approach the exercise with mindfulness. Pay attention to the spine's alignment, the deliberate activation of the lower body muscles, and the deliberate descent and ascent. By using mindfulness, the squat becomes a whole experience of strength and awareness rather than just a mechanical workout.

10. Humble Closure and Recuperation:

The Wall Squats conclude with a beautiful transition back to standing. Take a deep breath, letting go of the lower body muscles engaged, and purposefully stand up straight. A crucial element is the recovery phase, emphasizing a smooth transition from the squat to the standing posture. This deliberate ending improves the exercise's overall efficacy and fluidity.

The following are some advantages of wall squats:

1. **Lower Body Strength:** Wall squats strengthen the lower body by working the quadriceps, hamstrings, and glutes.
2. **Spinal Support:** The wall supports the lower back throughout the squat and encourages a neutral spine.
3. **Core Engagement:** Stability and a solid foundation are facilitated by activating the core muscles.
4. **Adaptable for All Levels:** Wall Squats are a versatile exercise that can be modified to suit various fitness levels.
5. **Mind-Body Connection:** The deliberate interaction and movement promote a stronger mind-body bond.
6. **Muscle Toning:** The lower body is sculpted and toned due to the deliberate activation of muscles.
7. **Stability and Confidence:** The wall's presence provides stability and confidence, enabling a concentrated squat.
8. **Breath Awareness:** Coordinated breathing improves awareness and maintains the squat's rhythmic flow.
9. **Safe and Effective Exercise:** The support of the wall makes the squat a safe exercise that engages muscles effectively without losing balance.
10. **Foundation for Further Progression:** The Pilates repertory includes a series of lower body exercises that build upon one another. Wall squats are an example of this fundamental activity.

Wall Squats are a fundamental exercise in the elegant choreography of Wall Pilates; they're a symphony of lower body strength, deliberate climb, and controlled fall. The squat becomes a canvas on which strength and stability are molded with deliberate movements as the body connects with the wall's support. Wall Squats are a powerful exercise that changes practitioners of all fitness levels because they perfectly combine muscular activation, breath awareness, and mindful presence.

3.2: Standing Leg Circles

A fascinating workout from the world of Wall Pilates, Standing Leg Circles reveals the secret to developing lower body strength, control, and flexibility. This exercise, rooted in Pilates principles, smoothly combines powerful leg motions with the wall's supporting direction. Join us as we explore the nuances of Standing Leg Circles and how they improve lower body mobility, strengthen the mind-muscle connection, and create a feeling of fluidity within the Pilates paradigm.

1. Starting the Circles of Standing Legs:

To begin the Standing Leg Circles, place your heels a few inches from the baseboard while standing with your side against the wall. With the wall acting as a solid anchor for the upper body, you can concentrate on the deft leg motions. Flex the foot and raise one leg laterally so that it is in line with the hip. The dynamic study of leg circles begins with this first stance.

2. Core Engagement and Alignment:

As you elevate the leg laterally, give careful alignment priority. The body should remain straight from head to heel without leaning or bending. Establish a solid base using your core muscles, especially your transverse abdominis. The alignment and core engagement promote regulated movement and minimize needless lower back strain.

3. Controlled Circular Motion:

The ability to perform circular leg motions with control and accuracy is the key to standing leg circles. With the leg up, draw little circles to explore the range of motion. The hip joint produces a regulated circular motion that highlights the activation of the hip flexors and abductors. By acting as a point of reference, the wall makes it possible to concentrate on the complex circles without worrying about balance.

4. Breath as a Mind-Body Connection:

In Standing Leg Circles, the mind-body connection is facilitated by the use of breath. Please take a deep breath to prepare for the circular action, then release it as you move your leg in the circles. The coordinated breathing strengthens awareness and maintains the movement's smoothness. As the leg glides around the circular pattern, the breath acts as a rhythmic guide, encouraging control and elegance.

5. Range of Motion and Flexibility of the Legs:

The exercise increases the range of motion in the hip joint and improves flexibility as the leg makes circles. The dynamic action enhances flexibility and mobility by actively activating the hip-circumferential muscles. A feeling of release is created in the hip joint by deliberately investigating the leg's range of motion.

6. Smooth Directional Transition:

Make a smooth transition to circles in the other way after investigating circles in one direction. To preserve the integrity of the movement, direction changes should be regulated and seamless. The dynamic shift improves total hip joint mobility by providing varied demands to the hip muscles. The workout has a rhythmic flow because of the fluid transition.

7. Extension and Flexion of the Foot:

Stepping foot flexion and extension into Standing Leg Circles adds another level of intricacy. Point and flex the foot alternately while the leg travels in a circular motion. This slight motion activates the calf muscles and improves ankle joint mobility. Using foot flexion and extension enhances the exercise's dynamic component and fosters overall lower limb strength and mobility.

8. Wall Support and Core Stability:

Keep your core stable during Standing Leg Circles to provide dynamic leg motions with a strong base. The wall lets you focus on perfecting the leg circles by giving the upper body a supporting anchor. The combination of wall support and core stability fosters an atmosphere conducive to precision and control.

9. Conscious Attention to Hip Muscles:

During Standing Leg Circles, pay close attention to how your hip muscles are used. Feel the hip abductors contracting as the leg goes laterally and the hip flexors activating as the leg elevates. By improving the mind-muscle link, this conscious awareness makes it possible to explore circular motion more deliberately and subtly.

10. Humble Closure and Recuperation:

With elegance and focus, drop the raised leg as you finish the Standing Leg Circles. Take a deep breath, relax your hip muscles, and stand back up in a neutral stance. An essential exercise component is the recovery period, which highlights the need for deliberate recuperation and the dynamic challenge. This intentional finish adds to the movement's overall charm.

The advantages of standing leg circles

1. **Enhanced Hip Flexibility:** By aggressively engaging the hip joint, standing leg circles help to promote more mobility and flexibility.

2. **Enhanced Hip Joint Stability**: The regulated circular motion strengthens and challenges the abductors and hip flexors, which improves joint stability.

3. **Mind-Body Connection:** Careful attention to hip muscles and coordinated breathing strengthen the mind-body connection.

4. **Dynamic Leg Articulation:** Including foot flexion and extension gives an emotional touch that improves ankle and leg articulation.

5. **Lower Body Strength:** The exercise improves general strength by using muscles across the lower body.

6. **Regulated Range of Motion:** The controlled movement inside the circular pattern fosters a refined and regulated range of motion.

7. **Adaptable for Varied Levels**: Standing Leg Circles are flexible enough to meet various fitness levels and objectives.

8. **Supportive Wall Anchor:** The wall acts as a stabilizing element, supporting the upper body and enabling the practitioner to concentrate on leg motions.

9. **Fluidity and elegance:** The exercise feels fluidity and elegance because of the regulated transitions and rhythmic circular movements.

10. **Artistic Integration of Movement:** Combining strength, flexibility, and control, Standing Leg Circles are a prime example of the Pilates paradigm's artistic movement integration.

Standing Leg Circles become a fluid dance in Wall Pilates' elegant choreography, a beautiful investigation of the lower body's flexibility, strength, and control. The exercise demonstrates the perfect fusion of movement and consciousness as the leg circles against the wall supporting the background. In Pilates, Standing Leg Circles allow practitioners to go on a dynamic exploratory voyage that shapes a harmonious connection between body and soul.

3.3: Wall Lunges

In Wall Pilates, Wall Lunges are a powerful and dynamic workout that combines lower body strength and stability. Based on Pilates principles, this exercise combines the wall's supporting direction with the deliberate movement of lunges. Let's dissect Wall Lunges, seeing how they work the lower body, improve balance, and cultivate a conscious relationship between breath and movement in the context of Pilates.

1. Starting Vertical Jumps:

Wall Lunges are started by placing your feet hip-width apart and your back against the wall. In addition to providing a solid base, the initial stance lays the groundwork for a deliberate drop into the lunge. Step forward with one foot, keeping enough space between your legs so that your knee and ankle will line up when you complete the lunge. The wall acts as a stable base and reference point for body alignment.

2. Core Engagement and Alignment:

In Wall Lunges, alignment is crucial. Ensure the front knee remains above the ankle as you lower yourself into the lunge, not extending beyond the toes. To establish a solid base, contract your core muscles simultaneously, such as the transverse abdominis and pelvic floor. The alignment and core engagement promote regulated movement and minimize needless lower back strain.

3. Continuous Descent and Ascent:

The deliberate fall and rise is what makes Wall Lunges so unique. As you bring your body down toward the floor, maintain your alignment and bend your front knee to a 90-degree angle. The quadriceps, hamstrings, and glutes are worked during the deliberate descent. Concentrate on driving the action via the engaged muscles to ensure a smooth and controlled transition as you return to the beginning position. Because the wall provides steady support, you can focus on the quality of the lunge rather than worrying about your balance.

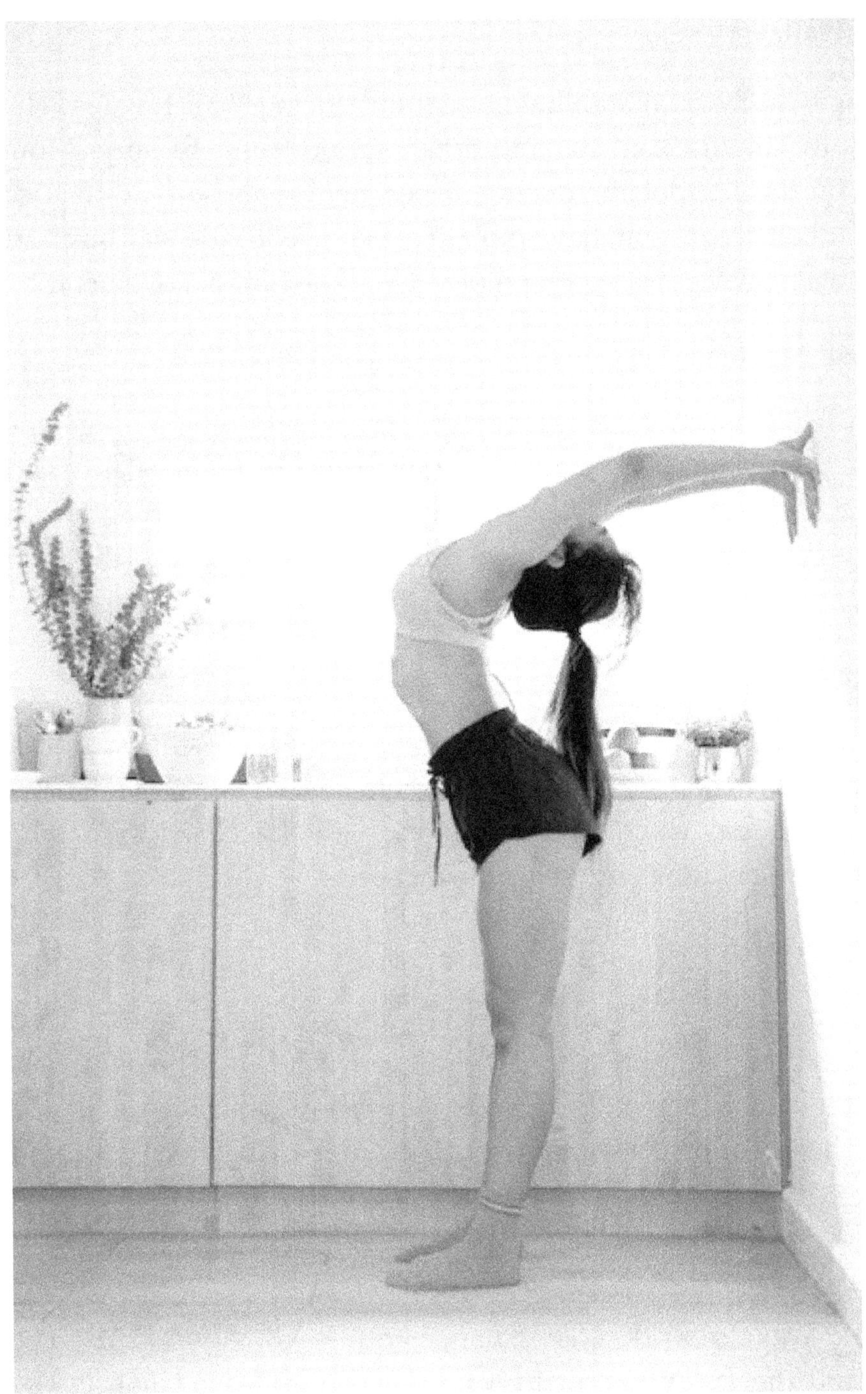

4. Breathing in Time with Movement:

In Wall Lunges, breath becomes the controlling principle. As you prepare to descend into the lunge, take a deep breath and stretch your rib cage. As you fall into the lunge, release your air and contract your core. Coordinated breathing strengthens awareness and maintains the movement's deliberate flow. The breath helps create a conscious link between movement and breathing by providing a regular cadence.

5. Supporting Stabilizing Wall:

The wall provides the upper body with stabilizing support during Wall Lunges. The hands may be placed lightly on the wall for additional support and balance. More stability is made possible by this supporting anchor, especially for those who may be attempting to improve their balance or who have mobility issues. With the wall support providing stability, practitioners may concentrate on perfecting the lunge movement.

6. Pay Attention to the Front and Back Legs:

When doing Wall Lunges, focus on your front and rear legs. When doing a lunge, the front leg works the glutes, hamstrings, and quadriceps. The back leg offers balance and stability at the same time. Activating both leg muscles enhances the strength and balance of the lower body. The activity is approached holistically, thanks to the dual emphasis.

7. Differences for the Progressive Task:

There are versions of wall lunges to suit varying fitness levels and objectives. Add a pulsating motion at the bottom of the lunge or carry weights in each hand to intensify the exercise. The range of action may be changed to suit individual needs or those who want a milder approach; this can be done with regular practice.

8. Mindful Transition between Lunges:

Perform Wall Lunges, making a conscious movement as you release each one. Keep your core engaged and your body aligned as you switch between legs. The deliberate transition guarantees that every lunge is performed precisely, which adds to the exercise's overall efficacy. The intentional motion strengthens the link between the mind and body.

9. Improving Balance and Coordination:

Wall lunges are a dynamic way to work your balance and coordination skills. The regulated climb, descent, and the wall's stabilizing support help improve balance. The front and rear legs work together to create a fluid movement that improves body awareness in general.

10. Humble Closure and Recuperation:

Wall Lunges must be finished with a graceful return to the starting position. Take a deep breath, letting go of the lower body muscles engaged, and purposefully stand up straight. The recovery phase is a crucial element that highlights the significance of deliberate recovery and the dynamic challenge. This thoughtful ending enhances the exercise's overall coherence and efficacy.

Wall lunges provide the following benefits:

1. **Lower Body Strength:** By focusing on the quadriceps, hamstrings, and glutes, wall lunges develop lower body strength.
2. **Balance Enhancement:** Because the wall provides stabilizing support, balance is improved, and the workout suits a range of fitness levels.
3. **Core Engagement:** The activation of the core muscles maintains total body alignment and offers a firm base for the lunge.
4. **Mind-Body Connection:** The focused concentration on alignment and coordinated breathing strengthens the mind-body connection.
5. **Progressive Challenge:** Variations support varying fitness levels and objectives by enabling advanced challenges.
6. **Stabilizing Wall Support:** The wall acts as a stabilizing element, giving assurance and control over the execution process.
7. **Improving Coordination:** Switching up your leg movements improves Coordination and increases body awareness in general.
8. **Adaptable for Varying Fitness Levels:** Wall Lunges are flexible enough to allow for adjustments to suit varying fitness levels.
9. **Fluidity and Control:** The steady wall support and the managed descent and climb help to create a feeling of fluidity and control.
10. **Foundation for Functional Mobility:** Wall Lunges are an excellent exercise that leads to better functional mobility, making everyday tasks more supported and efficient.

Wall Lunges become a dynamic movement in the elegant choreography of Wall Pilates, a symphony of lower body power, deliberate climb, and controlled fall. The lunge becomes a canvas on which strength and stability are molded with deliberate movements as the body connects with the wall's support. Wall Lunges are a transforming experience for practitioners of all fitness levels because they perfectly capture the Pilates journey's mindfulness, presence, breath awareness, and muscular engagement.

3.4: Inner Thigh Press

The Inner Thigh Press is a beautiful addition to the Wall Pilates repertory, revealing the secret to building elegant power and flexibility in the inner thighs. This exercise, rooted in Pilates principles, skillfully blends focused muscle activation with the wall's supporting embrace. Come along as we explore the nuances of the Pilates method's Inner Thigh Press, which tones the inner thigh muscles, increases flexibility, and creates a harmonious mind-body connection.

1. Starting the Inner Thigh Press:

Place your side against the wall to begin the Inner Thigh Press. Place yourself so the baseboard is a few inches away from your heels. Flex the foot and raise one leg laterally so that it is in line with the hip. By giving your upper body a solid anchor, the wall lets you focus on the deliberate motions of your inner thighs. This first alignment prepares the body for the elegant investigation of internal thigh involvement.

2. Core Engagement and Alignment:

As you elevate the leg laterally, give careful alignment priority. The body should remain straight from head to heel without leaning or bending. To establish a solid base, contract your core muscles, such as the transverse abdominis and pelvic floor. The alignment and core engagement promote regulated movement and minimize needless lower back strain.

3. Inner Thigh Controlled Engagement:

The deliberate activation of the inner thigh muscles is the fundamental component of the inner thigh press. To start, lightly push the elevated leg against the wall to activate the inner thigh muscles. You can feel the resistance when you go against the wall because it acts as a reference point. The deliberate activation of the inner thighs enhances the strength and flexibility of this sometimes overlooked muscle area.

4. Variations and Dynamic Movement:

Gently pulse the leg against the wall to explore dynamic movement inside the Inner Thigh Press. The dynamic feature of the pulsating action increases the intensity of the inner thigh muscle activation. Variations may be added to create a more challenging exercise, such as adjusting the leg's angle or the pulse rate. These variants provide flexibility by accommodating varying levels of fitness and objectives.

5. Breath as a Mind-Body Connection:

Inner Thigh Press uses breath as a channel for the mind-body connection. Breathe deeply, opening your rib cage as you prepare for the engagement. Completely release your breath as you force your leg against the wall, using your inner thigh muscles. The coordinated breathing strengthens awareness and maintains the movement's smoothness. Throughout the exercise, the breath is a rhythmic guide, encouraging control and elegance.

6. Extension and Flexion of the Foot:

Inserting foot flexion and extension into the Inner Thigh Press adds another difficulty level. Alternate between pointing and flexing the foot as you push the leg against the wall. This slight motion activates the calf muscles and improves ankle joint mobility. Using foot flexion and extension enhances the exercise's dynamic component and fosters flexibility and strength throughout the lower limb.

7. Supporting Stabilizing Wall:

The wall stabilizes the upper body during the Inner Thigh Press exercise. The hands may be placed lightly on the wall for additional support and balance. More stability is made possible by this supporting anchor, especially for those who may be attempting to improve their balance or who have mobility issues. With the wall support providing stability, practitioners can concentrate on honing the inner thigh engagement without worrying about losing their balance.

8. Concerned Attention to Inner Thigh Muscles:

Throughout the Inner Thigh Press, maintain a conscious concentration on activating the inner thigh muscles. The mu adductors, the muscles that pull the leg toward the body's midline, should be felt activating. By improving the mind-muscle connection, this conscious awareness makes it possible to explore inner thigh involvement more deliberately and subtly.

9. Improving Flexibility and Balance:

The inner thigh press aggressively works the muscles in the inner thighs responsible for flexibility and balance. The deliberate activation of these muscles results in increased balance and flexibility. The exercise develops a feeling of fluidity in the movement by gently exploring the inner thigh muscles' strength and suppleness.

10. Humble Closure and Recuperation:

The last step of the Inner Thigh Press is a seamless transition back to a neutral standing posture. With a deep breath, release the inner thigh muscles' engagement and intentionally descend the raised leg. The recovery phase is a crucial element that highlights the significance of deliberate recovery and the dynamic challenge. This thoughtful ending enhances the exercise's overall coherence and efficacy.

Inner thigh strength is enhanced with the Inner Thigh Press, which targets the adductor muscles, giving the inner thighs more strength.

1. **Flexibility Enhancement:** The deliberate activation encourages the inner thigh muscles to become more flexible, which improves the range of motion.

2. **Balance Improvement:** Because the wall provides stabilizing support, balance is improved, and the workout suits a range of fitness levels.

3. **Mind-Body Connection:** Careful attention to inner thigh engagement and coordinated breathing strengthen the mind-body connection.

4. **Dynamic Movement:** Foot flexion/extension and pulse changes offer an active element that increases engagement and strengthens the lower limbs.

5. **Adaptable for Varied Fitness Levels:** The Inner Thigh Press is flexible enough to adjust to suit varying fitness levels.

6. **Stabilizing Wall Support:** The wall stabilizes, giving confidence and control over the execution process.

7. **Fluidity and Control:** The exercise feels fluid and controlled because of the deliberate motions and regulated participation.

8. **Balance and Flexibility Enhancement:** The Inner Thigh Press works the muscles in the inner thighs responsible for balance and flexibility, encouraging a well-rounded combination of strength and flexibility.

9. **The basis for Inner Thigh Awareness:** The Inner Thigh Press is an activity that prepares the inner thigh muscles for future development in Pilates practice by increasing awareness and strength.

Inner Thigh Press becomes a sophisticated exercise in Wall Pilates' elegant choreography, a balletic investigation of inner thigh power, deliberate elegance, and controlled engagement. The exercise demonstrates the smooth transition between strength and flexibility in the Pilates method as the leg pushes against the wall supporting the background. In Pilates, Inner Thigh Press encourages practitioners to go on a dynamic exploratory voyage that shapes a harmonious relationship between body and soul.

3.5: Calf Raises with Wall Support

A sophisticated exercise in Wall Pilates, Calf Raises with Wall Support reveals the technique of elegantly and precisely shaping lower leg strength. This exercise, which has its roots in Pilates concepts, skillfully blends the wall's supporting direction with the regulated action of Calf raises. Let's take a closer look at the nuances of Calf Raises with Wall Support and see how this Pilates technique develops ankle mobility, strengthens the calves, and creates a balanced relationship between strength and stability.

1. Starting Calf Lifts with Wall Assistance:

With your feet hip-width apart, start Calf raises with wall support by standing with your hands gently resting on the wall. By giving your upper body a solid anchor, the wall frees up your attention so you can concentrate on the deliberate motions of your lower legs. This starting posture prepares the body for intentionally lifting the heels to target the calves muscles.

2. Core Engagement and Alignment:

As you raise your heels off the ground, prioritize careful alignment. Ankles, knees, and hips should all align as the body should remain straight from the head to the heels. Establish a solid base using your core muscles, especially your transverse abdominis. The alignment and core engagement promote regulated movement and minimize needless lower back strain.

3. Calf Raises with Contours:

The controlled heel lift is the key to Calf raises with wall support. Push through the balls of your feet and raise your heels off the floor. Pay close attention to your calf muscles, especially your gastrocnemius and soleus. Targeted muscle activation is encouraged since the movement is regulated, and the calves are the primary elevation source.

4. Variations and Dynamic Movement:

Try experimenting with different versions to see how Calf Raises moves dynamically. I suggest pulsing at its peak to further activate the calf muscles during the lift. For a more challenging version, try single-leg calf lifts as well. These variants provide flexibility, accommodating varying degrees of fitness and permitting more complex tasks.

5. Breath in Time with Movement:

The principle of Calf Raises with Wall Support is on breath. Take a deep breath to extend the rib cage and prepare for the Calf lift. As you raise your heels and contract your core, release the whole breath. The coordinated breathing strengthens awareness and maintains the movement's smoothness. Throughout the exercise, the breath is a rhythmic guide, encouraging control and elegance.

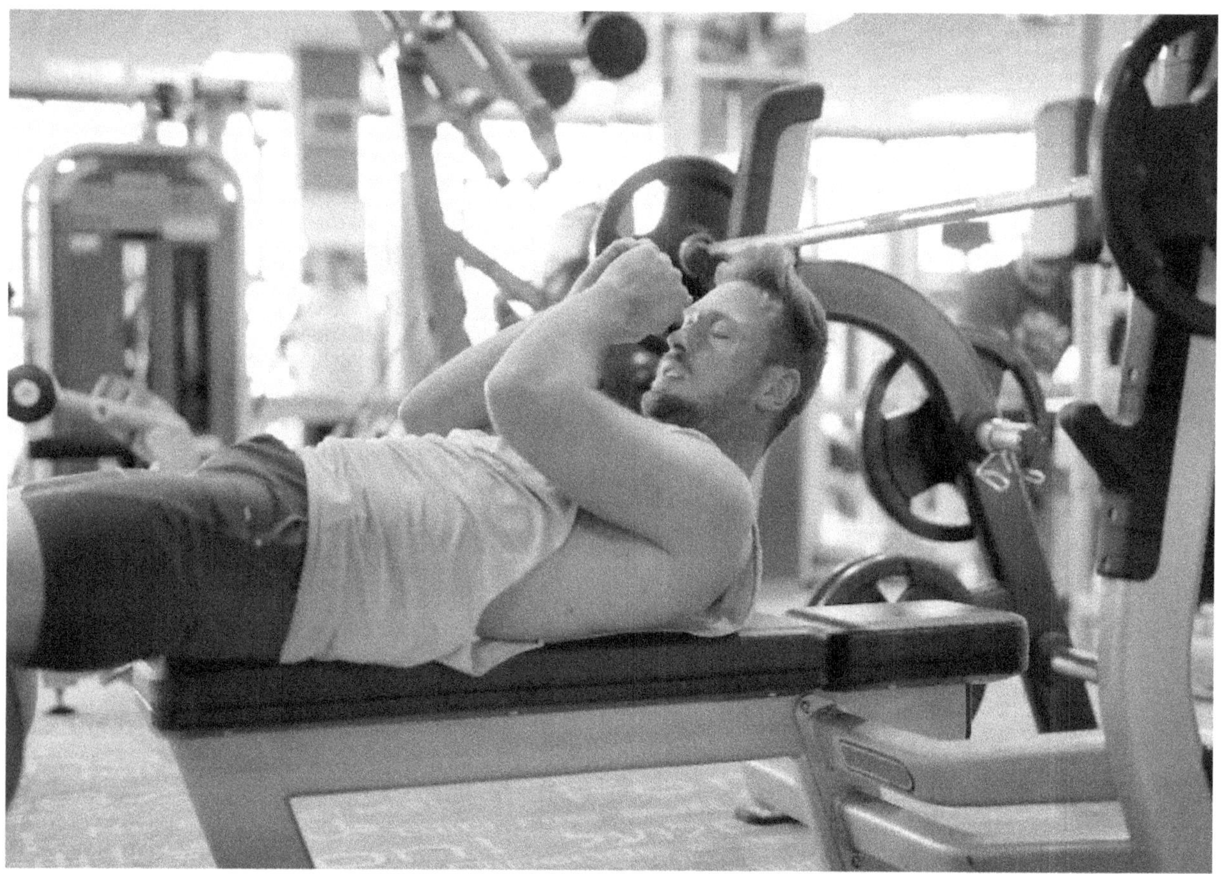

6. Articulation of the Foot:

By adjusting foot placement, you may add foot articulation to Calf raises. Start with raising the heels while the toes are pointed straight forward. Next, experiment with variations by turning the toes slightly inward and outward. This gentle motion works for many calf muscle groups, increasing overall ankle mobility and calf strength. The use of foot movement gives the workout an additional dynamic component.

7. Supporting Stabilizing Wall:

The wall provides the upper body with stabilizing support during Calf Raises. The hands may be placed lightly on the wall for additional support and balance. This supporting anchor makes Increased stability possible, especially for those who may be focusing on balancing out or managing issues with ankle movement. With the wall support providing stability, practitioners can concentrate on perfecting the heel elevation without worrying about losing their balance.

8. Concerned Attention to Calf Muscles:

Pay close attention to how the calf muscles contract during Calf raises. Feel the contraction of the more significant calf muscle, the gastrocnemius, and the deeper calf muscle, the soleus. By improving the mind-muscle connection, this conscious awareness makes it possible to explore calf muscle involvement more deliberately and subtly.

9. Improving Ankle Mobility and Balance:

Exercises incorporating Wall Support for Calf Raises aggressively work the muscles related to ankle mobility and balance. The deliberate elevation of the heels tests the ankle joint's stabilizing muscles. The exercise develops a feeling of fluidity in the movement by gently exploring the calves' strength and mobility.

10. Humble Closure and Recuperation:

The last step in Calf Raises is a beautiful landing back on your feet. Breathe deeply, letting go of the calf muscles' engagement and deliberately bringing the heels down. The recovery phase is a crucial element that highlights the significance of deliberate recovery and the dynamic challenge. This thoughtful ending enhances the exercise's overall coherence and efficacy.

Advantages of Wall-Supported Calf Raises:

1. **Calf Muscle Strengthening:** Calf Raises strengthen the calves by focusing on the gastrocnemius and soleus muscles.

2. **Improving Ankle Stability**: The deliberate motion strains the muscles in charge of maintaining the stability of the ankle joint, which enhances stability.

3. **Balance Improvement:** Because the wall provides stabilizing support, balance is improved, and the workout suits a range of fitness levels.

4. **Mind-Body Connection:** The attentive attention to engaging the calf muscles and the coordinated breathing enhances the mind-body connection.

5. **Dynamic Movement:** To enhance engagement and build general lower leg strength, emotional components like foot articulation, single-leg rises, and pulsing variants are included.

6. **Adaptable for Varied Fitness Levels:** Wall-supported Calf raises are versatile, allowing adjustments to suit a range of fitness levels.

7. **Stabilizing Wall Support:** The wall stabilizes, giving confidence and control over the execution process.

8. **Fluidity and Control:** The workout feels fluidity and control because of the deliberate motions and controlled ascent.

9. **Improving Ankle Mobility and Balance:** Calf raises aggressively work the muscles related to ankle mobility and balance, encouraging a well-balanced combination of strength and flexibility.

10. **Basis for Lower Leg Awareness:** Calf Raises with Wall Support is an essential Pilates exercise that strengthens and increases calves' awareness, laying the groundwork for further advancement in the technique.

Calf Raises with Wall Support become a poised movement in the elegant dance of Wall Pilates, a symphony of lower leg strength, controlled elevation, and deliberate elegance. The exercise becomes a testimony to the seamless integration of strength and stability within the Pilates journey as the heels rise against the supporting background of the wall. In the domain of Pilates, Calf Raises with Wall Support encourages practitioners to go on a dynamic exploratory voyage that shapes a harmonious relationship between body and soul.

3.6: Glute Kickbacks

Glute Kickbacks are a refined and focused movement from the Wall Pilates repertoire, revealing the secret to building strength and definition in the glutes. This exercise, rooted in Pilates principles, skillfully blends controlled leg motions with the wall's supporting direction. Let's tour the nuances of Glute Kickbacks, learn how they tone the gluteal muscles, improve hip flexion, and cultivate a balanced relationship between grace and strength within the Pilates model.

1. Starting Glute Reactions:

With your hands softly resting on the wall, face the wall to begin Glute Kickbacks. Ensure your spine is neutral and your feet are hip-width apart. This starting position lays the foundation for the deliberate leg motions that will work the glutes. By providing a stable anchor for the upper body, the wall enables you to concentrate on the intentional activation of your glute muscles.

2. Core Engagement and Alignment:

Pay attention to your alignment as you slowly raise one leg behind you. The body should remain straight from head to heel, with the hips aligned against the wall. Establish a solid base using your core muscles, especially your transverse abdominis. The alignment and core engagement promote regulated movement and minimize needless lower back strain.

3. Regulated Glute Engagement:

Controlled activation of the glute muscles is the key to Glute Kickbacks. Concentrate on tightening your glutes to start the action as you raise your leg behind you. Using the wall as a reference point, you can feel the resistance as you push your leg back. The deliberate activation of the glutes adds to this vital muscle group's strength and definition.

4. Variations and Dynamic Movement:

Investigate Glute Kickbacks' dynamic movement by adding variants. To increase the activation of the glute muscles, think about pulsing at the peak of the kickback. For a more challenging exercise, consider varying the pace or angle at which you do the leg lift. These variants provide flexibility, accommodating varying degrees of fitness and permitting more complex tasks.

5. Breath in Time with Movement:

Glute Kickbacks turn breathing into a compass. As you prepare for the kickback, take a deep breath and extend your rib cage. Fully exhale as you raise your leg, activating your core muscles and paying attention to your glutes contracting. The coordinated breathing strengthens awareness and maintains the movement's smoothness. Throughout the exercise, the breath is a rhythmic guide, encouraging control and elegance.

6. Extension and Flexion of the Foot:

By adding changes in foot posture, Glute Kickbacks may include foot flexion and extension. Try flexing the foot as you drop the leg and pointing the toes during the kickback. This slight motion increases general hip mobility by activating several gluteal muscles. The workout gains a dynamic aspect by including foot flexion and extension.

7. Supporting Stabilizing Wall:

The wall provides the upper body with stabilizing support during Glute Kickbacks. The hands may be placed lightly on the wall for additional support and balance. More stability is made possible by this supporting anchor, especially for those who may be attempting to improve their balance or who have mobility issues. With the wall support providing stability, practitioners can concentrate on honing their glute engagement without worrying about losing their balance.

8. Concerned Attention to Glute Muscles:

Pay close attention to how the glute muscles contract during glute kickbacks. During the kickback, notice how the most excellent glute muscle, the gluteus maximus, contracts. By improving the mind-muscle connection, this conscious awareness makes it possible to explore glute muscle involvement more deliberately and subtly.

9. Improving Hip Mobility and Balance:

Glute Kickbacks work the muscles responsible for hip mobility and balance. The muscles that stabilize the hip joint are put to the test by the deliberate lifting of the leg. The exercise develops a feeling of fluidity in the action by gently exploring the glutes' strength and mobility.

10. Humble Closure and Recuperation:

Glute Kickbacks end with a seamless transition back to a neutral standing stance. With purpose, drop the raised leg after taking a deep breath and letting go of the glute muscles' engagement. The recovery phase is a crucial element that highlights the significance of deliberate recovery and the dynamic challenge. This thoughtful ending enhances the exercise's overall coherence and efficacy.

Glute Kickback Benefits:

1. **Strengthening of the Gluteal Muscle:** Glute Kickbacks work the gluteus maximus, which gives the glutes more definition and strength.

2. **Improved Hip Mobility:** Deliberate motion strains the muscles, maintaining the hip joint and enhancing hip mobility.

3. **Balance Improvement:** Because the wall provides stabilizing support, balance is improved, and the workout suits a range of fitness levels.

4. **Mind-Body Connection:** The focus on engaging the glute muscles and the coordinated breathing strengthens the mind-body connection.

5. **Dynamic Movement:** Different angles, foot flexion/extension, and pulsing variations offer emotional components that heighten engagement and enhance gluteal strength overall.

6. **Adaptable for Varied Fitness Levels:** Glute Kickbacks may be modified to meet the needs of individuals with varying fitness levels.

7. **Stabilizing Wall Support:** The wall stabilizes, giving confidence and control over the execution process.

8. **Fluidity and Control:** The workout has a sensation of fluidity and control because of the deliberate motions and controlled kickback.

9. **Balance and Hip Mobility Enhancement:** Glute Kickbacks intensively work the muscles that support hip mobility and balance, encouraging a well-balanced combination of strength and flexibility.

10. **The basis for Gluteal Awareness:** Glute Kickbacks function as a fundamental exercise that strengthens and increases glute awareness, laying the groundwork for further Pilates practice advancement.

Glute Kickbacks are a sophisticated exercise that explores gluteal power, controlled lift, and deliberate elegance in the elegant choreography of Wall Pilates. The exercise shows how power and grace can be combined effortlessly in the Pilates method as the leg stretches against the wall supporting surface. Within the Pilates domain, Glute Kickbacks encourage practitioners to go on a dynamic exploratory voyage that shapes a harmonious connection between body and soul.

3.7: Pilates Wall Chair

Within the realm of Wall Pilates, the Pilates Wall Chair is a unique and transformational workout that offers a symphony of controlled motions that enhance lower body strength with functional accuracy. Based on Pilates' fundamentals, this exercise skillfully combines strength, stability, and flexibility with the wall's supporting background. Let's examine the nuances of the Pilates Wall Chair and how, within the Pilates paradigm, it develops alignment, tones the lower body muscles, and creates a harmonic relationship between strength and functional movement.

1. Starting with the Pilates Wall Chair:

Place your back against the wall and your feet hip-width apart to begin the Pilates Wall Chair. With the wall acting as a structural support for the upper body, the Wall Chair mimics the shape of a sitting chair. This initial place transformation is the basis for transforming lower body motions that come next. Because the wall acts as a stabilizing anchor, you may focus on the deliberate activation of your lower body muscles.

2. Core Engagement and Alignment:

Ensure your body is aligned correctly as you descend into a sitting posture, simulating a chair. The lower back should be softly pressed against the wall while the spine remains neutral. To establish a solid base, contract your core muscles, such as the transverse abdominis and pelvic floor. The alignment and core engagement promote regulated movement and minimize needless lower back strain.

3. Continued Descending and Ascending:

The Pilates Wall Chair's deliberate lowering and raising motions are the core. Ensure your knees are over your ankles, and lower your body into a sitting posture. The quadriceps, hamstrings, and glutes are worked during the deliberate descent. To ensure a smooth and controlled transition, concentrate on driving the action with the engaged lower body muscles as you return to the beginning position. Because the wall offers constant support, you can focus on the movement's quality rather than worrying about your balance.

4. Variations and Dynamic Movement:

Investigate dynamic movement in the Pilates Wall Chair by adding tweaks. To increase the lower body muscular activation level, try adding pulses at the lowest point of the sitting posture. Adjusting the tempo of the exercises or adding little isometric holds are examples of variations that provide flexibility, accommodating varying degrees of fitness and permitting more complex tasks.

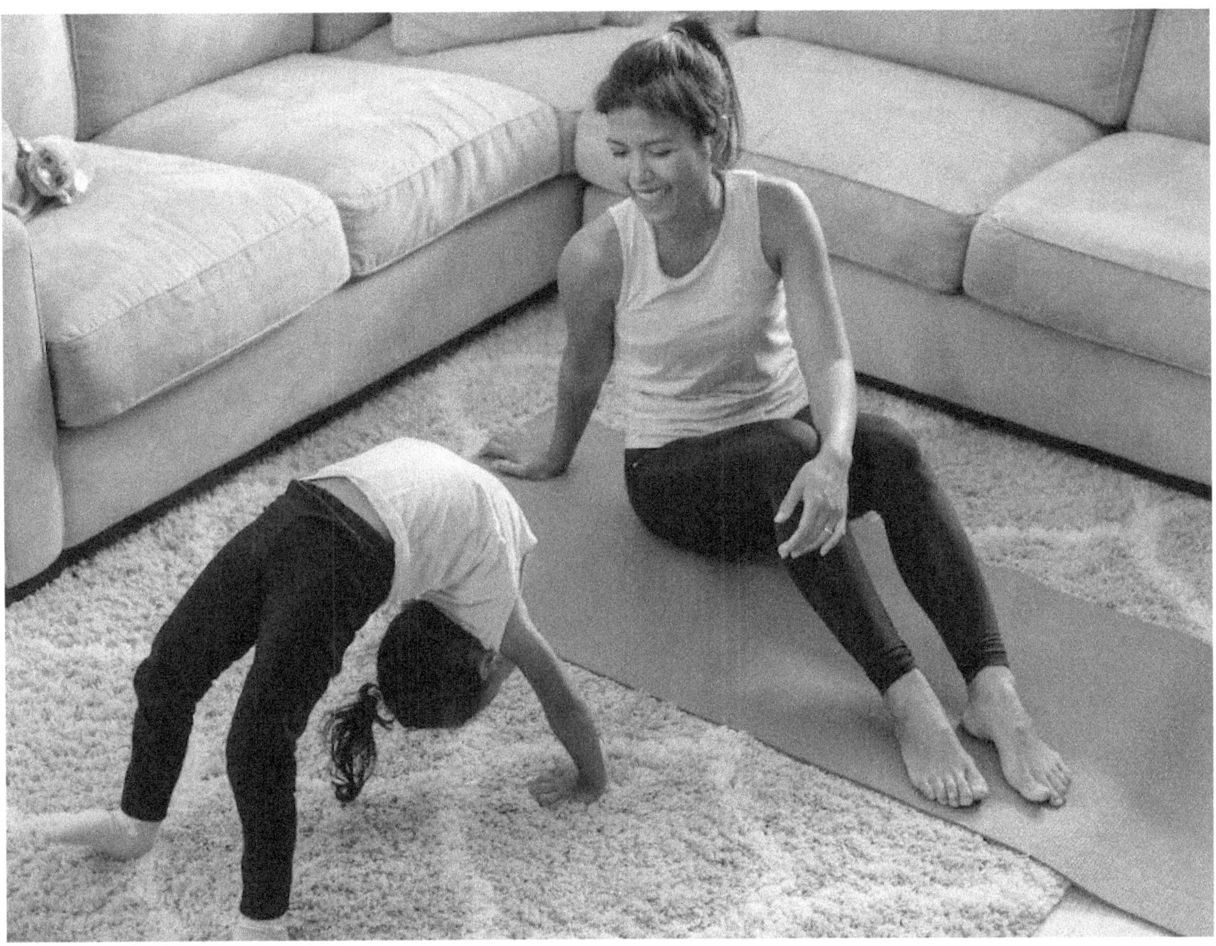

5. Breath in Time with Movement:

The Pilates Wall Chair starts to include breathing. As you are about to descend, take a deep breath and extend your rib cage. As you bring your body down to a sitting posture, release all your air and contract your core muscles. The coordinated breathing strengthens awareness and maintains the movement's smoothness. Throughout the exercise, the breath is a rhythmic guide, encouraging control and elegance.

6. Supporting Stabilizing Wall:

The wall stabilizes the upper body during the Pilates Wall Chair. The hands may be placed lightly on the wall for additional support and balance. More stability is made possible by this supporting anchor, especially for those who may be attempting to strengthen their lower body or improve their balance. Through the stabilizing wall support, practitioners may concentrate on honing the techniques without worrying about losing their equilibrium.

7. Concerned Attention to Lower Body Muscles:

Throughout the Pilates Wall Chair, maintain a careful concentration on the engaged lower body muscles. Feel your quadriceps, hamstrings, and glutes firing up as they cooperate to help you manage the rise and descent. By improving the mind-muscle link, this conscious awareness makes it possible to explore lower-body muscle activation more deliberately and subtly.

8. Alignment Verification and Adjustment:

Make sure your knees are in line with your ankles, and your spine stays neutral by periodically checking your alignment while doing the Pilates Wall Chair. The depth of the sitting posture may be changed to consider any physical limitations or individual fitness levels. Good form is stressed to get the most out of the workout and enhance its efficiency.

9. Integration of Functional Movement:

The Pilates Wall Chair incorporates functional motions beyond individual muscle activation. Because the seated posture resembles sitting on a chair, it's a valuable workout that may help with everyday tasks. Incorporating functional movement into the workout increases its applicability to daily life.

10. Humble Closure and Recuperation:

The Pilates Wall Chair concludes with a flowing transition back to standing. Take a deep breath, letting go of the lower body muscles engaged, and purposefully stand up straight. The recovery phase is a crucial element that highlights the significance of deliberate recovery and the dynamic challenge. This thoughtful ending enhances the exercise's overall coherence and efficacy.

Pilates Wall Chair Benefits:

1. **Development of Lower Body Strength:** The Pilates Wall Chair works the quadriceps, hamstrings, and glutes, developing lower body strength.
2. **Functional Movement Integration:** The exercise is relevant to everyday tasks since it replicates the motion of sitting in a chair.
3. **Balance Improvement:** Because the wall provides stabilizing support, balance is improved, and the workout suits a range of fitness levels.
4. **Mind-Body Connection:** The attentive attention to engaging the muscles in the lower body and the coordinated breathing strengthens the mind-body connection.
5. **Dynamic Movement:** Various pulse patterns and other dynamic exercises boost lower body strength overall and increase engagement.

6. **Adaptable for Varied Fitness Levels**: The Pilates Wall Chair may be modified to match a range of fitness levels thanks to its versatility.
7. **Stabilizing Wall Support:** The wall stabilizes, giving confidence and control over the execution process.
8. **Fluidity and Control:** The exercise has a sensation of fluidity and control because of the regulated fall and ascent and the stabilizing wall support.
9. **Alignment Focus:** This exercise strongly emphasizes alignment, encouraging optimum muscular activation and helps avoid putting too much tension on the lower back.
10. **Foundation for Functional Movement:** The Pilates Wall Chair is an activity that provides better functional movement, which enhances the efficiency and stability of everyday tasks.

The Pilates Wall Chair is a dynamic activity that combines controlled strength, functional accuracy, and purposeful elegance in Wall Pilates' elegant choreography. The exercise showcases how strength and functional movement seamlessly integrate into the Pilates journey as the body falls and ascends against the wall supporting background. The Pilates Wall Chair challenges users to go on a dynamic discovery trip, creating a balanced relationship between the body and the soul in the Pilates domain.

Chapter 4: Upper Body and Arm Toning

4.1: Wall Push-Ups

An essential exercise in wall Pilates, wall push-ups are an effective way to develop upper body strength with precise assistance. Using the wall's support to target the arms, chest, and shoulders, this Pilates-inspired workout targets major muscle groups. Let's examine the nuances of wall push-ups and see how, in the context of the Pilates paradigm, they develop strength, encourage attentive movement, and support a balanced relationship between the upper and lower body.

1. Starting Point:

Wall Push-Ups: Stand facing the wall with your feet hip-width apart to start. Place your hands slightly wider than shoulder-width apart on the wall at shoulder height. The body should create a straight line from the head to the heels, with the arms stretched to their maximum length. The wall provides a stabilizing support that permits the regulated activation of the muscles in the upper body.

2. Core Engagement and Alignment:

When doing Wall Push-Ups, ensure your body is in a straight line for optimal alignment. Establish a solid base using your core muscles, especially your transverse abdominis. The alignment and core engagement promote regulated movement and help avoid undue pressure on the lower back. This basic configuration is essential to maximize the exercise's efficacy.

3. Continuous Descent and Ascent:

The controlled motions on the climb and descent make a wall push-up. Bending your elbows, lower your body toward the wall while keeping your head and heels straight. As you drop, concentrate on using your arm, chest, and shoulder muscles. Using the power of the upper body, push away from the wall in the controlled ascent. Targeted muscle regions are engaged mindfully and precisely thanks to this deliberate action.

4. Variations and Dynamic Movement:

Try adding modifications to Wall Push-Ups to explore dynamic movement. To enhance the involvement of the arms and chest, think about adding pulses at the bottom of the push-up. Changes in how one places their hands or feet may be flexible, accommodating varying degrees of fitness and enabling progressively more complex tasks. The wall support provides the ability to experiment with various angles and ranges of motion.

5. Breath in Time with Movement:

Taking deep breaths becomes crucial during Wall Push-Ups. As you are about to descend, take a deep breath and extend your rib cage. As you bring your body down toward the wall, release your air, contract your core, and concentrate on the deliberate action. The coordinated breathing strengthens awareness and maintains the movement's smoothness. It is a rhythmic guide, encouraging control and elegance in the activity.

6. Supporting Stabilizing Wall:

The wall provides the upper body with stabilizing support during Wall Push-Ups. The hands continue to be in touch with the wall, acting as a constant source of support. This supporting component benefits those trying to strengthen their upper bodies or who may have wrist problems. With the wall support providing stability, practitioners can concentrate on honing the technique without worrying about losing their balance.

7. Conscientious Attention to Upper Body Muscles:

Throughout Wall Push-Ups, pay close attention to how your upper body muscles are used. Feel your shoulders, triceps, and chest activating as they cooperate to manage the rise and descent. By improving the mind-muscle link, this conscious awareness makes it possible to explore upper-body muscle activation more deliberately and subtly.

8. Alignment Verification and Adjustment:

Throughout Wall Push-Ups, periodically check your alignment to make sure your body stays in a straight line. Modifications may be made to suit varying degrees of fitness by running the push-up's angle or distance from the wall. The focus is on keeping the correct form to optimize the benefits of the exercise and reduce the chance of strain.

9. Building Upper Body Strength:

Wall Push-Ups are a great way to build upper body strength since they work the arms, chest, and shoulders muscles. Targeted muscle activation made possible by the deliberate movement adds to the region's improved strength and definition.

10. Humble Closure and Recuperation:

Wall Push-Ups conclude with an elegant stride away from the wall. Take a deep breath, letting go of the upper body muscles engaged, and purposefully stand up straight. The recovery phase is a crucial element that highlights the significance of deliberate recovery and the dynamic challenge. This thoughtful ending enhances the exercise's overall coherence and efficacy.

The following are some advantages of wall push-ups:

1. **Development of Upper Body Strength:** Wall push-ups work the muscles in the shoulders, chest, and arms, which promotes the development of upper body strength.
2. **Controlled Movement:** This exercise promotes precise and deliberate activation of the targeted muscle groups by emphasizing a controlled descent and ascent.
3. **Breath-Movement Synchronization:** Bringing awareness and the exercise's fluidity together, synchronized breath and movement contribute to a mindful Pilates practice.
4. **Stabilizing Wall Support:** The wall is a stabilizing force, supporting confident and controlled execution. This is especially helpful for those trying to strengthen their upper bodies.
5. **Mind-Body Connection:** By paying careful attention to the activation of upper body muscles, one may strengthen the mind-body connection and cultivate a feeling of grace and control during exercise.
6. **Adaptable for Varied Fitness Levels:** Wall push-ups are flexible enough to meet a range of fitness levels and allow for increasing difficulty.
7. **Alignment Emphasis:** The exercise emphasizes alignment to the fullest extent possible to maximize muscle activation and minimize needless lower back strain.
8. **Basis for Upper Body Awareness:** Wall Push-Ups are essential exercises that develop strength and awareness in the arms, chest, and shoulders muscles, laying the groundwork for further advancement in Pilates practice.

Wall Push-Ups are a fundamental action in the elegant choreography of Wall Pilates; they are an expressive demonstration of controlled strength, conscious engagement, and supporting accuracy. The exercise demonstrates how strength and mindful movement are seamlessly integrated into the Pilates journey as the body travels toward and away from the wall. Wall-Pushing Ups encourage practitioners to explore their bodies dynamically and create a harmonious body-spirit connection in the Pilates domain.

4.2: Tricep Dips using Wall

A specific exercise in Wall Pilates, wall-based tricep dips reveal the secret to precisely and steadily building arm strength. Based on Pilates principles, this exercise targets the triceps, or the muscles at the rear of the arms, by skillfully combining controlled motions with the support of the wall. Let's explore the nuances of wall-based Tricep Dips, including how they tone the triceps, improve arm definition, and create a harmonic relationship between strength and conscious movement within the framework of Pilates.

1. Starting Point:

Place your back against the wall while sitting on the floor to begin doing Tricep Dips. With your fingers pointing down, place your hands on the wall slightly wider than shoulder-width apart. Make a straight line from your head to your heels as you extend your legs. The wall supports the upper body and creates the ideal environment for deliberate actions that focus on the triceps.

2. Core Engagement and Alignment:

When doing Tricep Dips, ensure your back stays in touch with the wall to maintain good alignment. Establish a solid base using your core muscles, especially your transverse abdominis. The alignment and core engagement promote regulated movement and minimize needless lower back strain. This basic configuration is essential to maximize the exercise's efficacy.

3. Continuous Descent and Ascent:

The deliberate climb and descent motions are what make tricep dips so effective. Bend your elbows to point straight back as you lower your body toward the floor. As you drop, concentrate on using your triceps, the muscles at the rear of your arms. Using the power of your triceps, push away from the wall in this controlled ascent. This deliberate action engages The targeted muscle area mindfully and precisely.

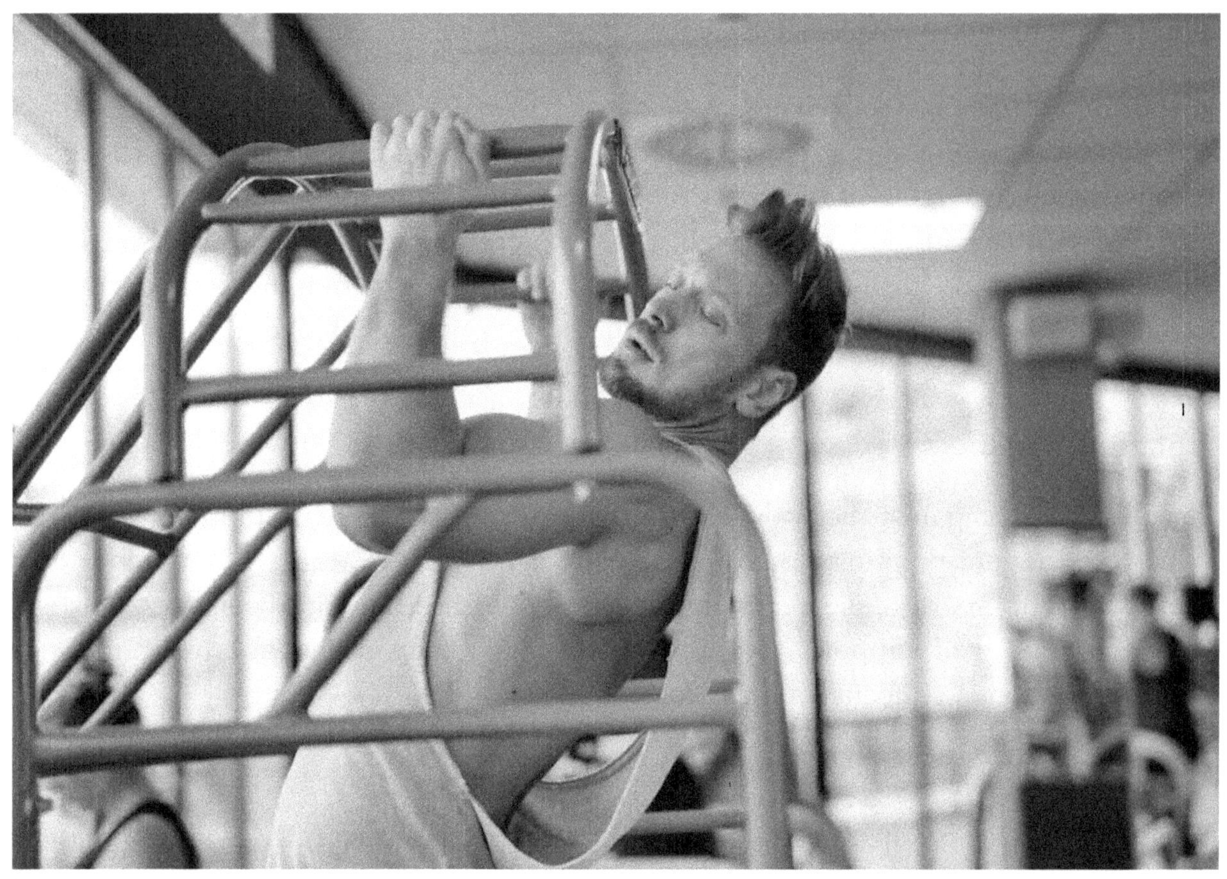

4. Variations and Dynamic Movement:

Try experimenting with different variants to discover dynamic movement in Tricep Dips. To increase the intensity of the triceps contraction, think about adding pulses at the bottom of the dip. Changes in how one places their hands or feet may be flexible, accommodating varying degrees of fitness and enabling progressively more complex tasks. Because of the wall support's versatility, you may try various angles and motion ranges.

5. Breath in Time with Movement:

Breath becomes an essential part of the Tricep Dip exercise. As you are about to descend, take a deep breath and extend your rib cage. As you bring your body down to the floor, release all your air while contracting your core and paying attention to the deliberate action. The coordinated breathing strengthens awareness and maintains the movement's smoothness. It is a rhythmic guide, encouraging control and elegance in the activity.

6. Supporting Stabilizing Wall:

The wall provides the upper body with stabilizing support during Tricep Dips. The hands continue to be in touch with the wall, acting as a constant source of support. This supporting component benefits those trying to strengthen their arms or who may have wrist problems. With the wall support providing stability, practitioners can concentrate on honing their moves without worrying about losing their balance.

7. Concise Attention to Triceps:

Pay close attention to your triceps while you do Tricep Dips. Since the activation of the back muscles of your arms as they cooperate to regulate the rise and descent. By improving the mind-muscle link, this conscious awareness makes it possible to explore tricep muscle activation more deliberately and subtly.

8. Alignment Verification and Adjustment:

Ensure your back touches the wall during Tricep Dips by periodically checking your alignment. Adjustments may be made to suit varying fitness levels by running the distance from the wall or the depth of the dip. The focus is on keeping the correct form to optimize the benefits of the exercise and reduce the chance of strain.

9. Building Arm Strength:

Arm strength is developed by the active activation of the triceps during Tricep Dips exercise. The precise muscle activation made possible by the regulated movement helps to define and strengthen the muscles in the back of the arms.

10. Humble Closure and Recuperation:

The last rep of a Tricep Dip is a fluid transition back to the beginning position. Sit straight with purpose after taking a deep breath and letting go of the triceps contraction. The recovery phase is a crucial element that highlights the significance of deliberate recovery and the dynamic challenge. This thoughtful ending enhances the exercise's overall coherence and efficacy.

Advantages of Wall Tricep Dips

1. **Tricep Strength Development:** By focusing on and activating the triceps, tricep dips help to build arm strength.

2. **Controlled Movement:** This exercise focuses on a deliberate and precise contraction and ascension of the triceps.

3. **Breath-Movement Synchronization:** Bringing awareness and the exercise's fluidity together, synchronized breath and movement contribute to a mindful Pilates practice.

4. **Stabilizing Wall Support:** The wall is a stabilizing force, supporting confident and controlled execution. This is especially helpful for those who are trying to strengthen their arms.

5. **Mind-Body Connection:** Paying close attention to activating the tricep muscles helps strengthen the mind-body connection, promoting control and grace throughout the exercise.

6. **Adaptable for Varied Fitness Levels**: Tricep dips are flexible enough to adjust to various fitness levels and allow for increasing difficulty.

7. **Alignment Emphasis:** The exercise emphasizes alignment to the fullest extent possible to maximize muscle activation and minimize needless lower back strain.

8. **Basis for Upper Body Awareness:** Tricep Dips are an essential exercise that develops the strength and awareness of the triceps, laying the groundwork for further advancement in Pilates practice.

Tricep Dips Using Wall become a shaping exercise in the elegant choreography of Wall Pilates, a rhythmic ballet of controlled strength, conscious engagement, and supporting accuracy. The exercise provides a testimony to the seamless integration of strength and mindful movement within the Pilates journey as the body falls and ascends against the supporting wall. Practitioners of Tricep Dips are invited to set off on a journey of In the Pilates domain, energetic inquiry shapes a healthy body-spirit relationship.

4.3: Wall Angels

Wall Angels is a heavenly exercise in the Wall Pilates repertoire that reveals how to shape shoulder mobility and stability precisely with an air of mystery. Based on Pilates principles, this exercise targets the complex muscles surrounding the shoulder blades by combining controlled motions with the wall's supporting direction. Let's investigate the nuances of Wall Angels, learning how they improve shoulder range of motion, stabilize the body, and keep a balanced relationship between strength and flowing movement in the context of the Pilates model.

1. Starting Point:

To begin Wall Angels, stand with your back to the wall and ensure that your head and tailbone are in touch with the wall and the complete spine. Place your feet a few inches from the wall and hip-width apart. Beginning at your sides, place your elbows 90 degrees bent and your backs on the wall to start the exercise. This first posture lays the groundwork for the subsequent deliberate motions, enabling the wall to provide encouraging direction.

2. Core Engagement and Alignment:

When doing Wall Angels, ensure your spine stays in touch with the wall the whole time to maintain appropriate alignment. Establish a solid base using your core muscles, especially your transverse abdominis. The alignment and core engagement promote regulated movement and minimize needless lower back strain. This basic configuration is essential to maximize the exercise's efficacy.

3. Managed Arm Motions:

The precise arm motions that imitate the flowing motion of an angel's wings make Wall Angels unique. Keeping the backs of your hands on the wall, slide your arms up the wall and out over your head. Concentrate on using the muscles around your shoulder blades as you extend your arms. Regaining your starting posture with your arms is part of the controlled descent. This deliberate action engages The targeted muscle area mindfully and precisely.

4. Variations and Dynamic Movement:

Try adding modifications to Wall Angels to explore dynamic movement. Add little pulses at the maximum Point of the arm extension to increase the intensity of the shoulder muscles being engaged. Changes in arm angles or hand placement may be flexible, accommodating varying degrees of fitness and permitting progressively more complex tasks. Because of the wall support's flexibility, you may try out various ranges of motion.

5. Breath in Time with Movement:

For Wall Angels, breathing turns into a compass. As you start the upward motion, take a deep breath and extend your rib cage. Fully exhale as you raise your arms over your head, utilizing your core to control the movement. The coordinated breathing strengthens awareness and supports the movement's smoothness. It is a rhythmic guide, encouraging control and elegance in the activity.

6. Supporting Stabilizing Wall:

The wall serves as the upper body's stabilizing support during Wall Angels. A constant anchor for stability is provided by the backs of the hands and the whole spine staying in touch with the wall. Those who are recuperating from shoulder injuries or seeking to improve shoulder mobility may particularly benefit from this supporting component. With the wall support providing stability, practitioners can concentrate on honing their moves without worrying about losing their balance.

7. Conscientious Attention to Shoulder Blades:

Throughout Wall Angels, pay close attention to how the muscles around your shoulder blades are used. As these muscles cooperate to govern the arm motions, feel them contracting. By improving the mind-muscle link, this conscious awareness makes it possible to explore shoulder blade muscle activation more deliberately and subtly.

8. Alignment Verification and Adjustment:

Throughout Wall Angels, ensure your whole spine stays in touch with the wall by periodically checking your alignment. To accommodate varying degrees of fitness, you may modify it by changing the range of motion or the angle at which your arms are held. The focus is on keeping the correct form to optimize the benefits of the exercise and reduce the chance of strain.

9. Improving Shoulder Mobility:

Wall Angels aggressively work the muscles that surround the shoulder blades, increasing their range of motion. The deliberate motions promote a more excellent range of motion by enabling a beautiful investigation of shoulder mobility.

10. Humble Closure and Recuperation:

Returning your arms to the beginning position is the last step in finishing wall angels. Take a deep breath, letting go of the shoulder muscles' engagement, and purposefully stand up straight. The recovery phase is a crucial element that highlights the significance of deliberate recovery and the dynamic challenge. This thoughtful ending enhances the exercise's overall coherence and efficacy.

Advantages of Wall Angels:

1. **Shoulder Mobility Enhancement:** Wall Angels actively work to improve the range of motion of the muscles that surround the shoulder blades.
2. **Controlled Movement:** This exercise focuses on deliberate and precise arm motions that impact the targeted shoulder muscles.

3. **Breath-Movement Synchronization:** Bringing awareness and the exercise's fluidity together, synchronized breath and movement contribute to a mindful Pilates practice.
4. **Stabilizing Wall Support:** The wall is a stabilizing force, supporting confident and controlled execution. This is especially helpful for those trying to improve their shoulder mobility.
5. **Mind-Body Connection:** Paying close attention to how the shoulder blade muscles engage strengthens the mind-body connection and promotes control and elegance in the exercise.
6. **Adaptable for Varying Fitness Levels:** Wall Angels are flexible, allowing for adjustments to suit varying fitness levels and space for escalating difficulties.
7. **Posture Emphasis:** The exercise focuses on keeping the body in the correct posture, encouraging the best possible muscle activation, and avoiding needless lower back strain.
8. **The basis for Shoulder Awareness:** Wall Angels function as an essential exercise that strengthens and increases awareness in the muscles that surround the shoulder blades, laying the groundwork for further Pilates practice advancement.

Wall Angels are a heavenly movement that arises in the elegant choreography of Wall Pilates. It is a dance of controlled power, focused participation, and supporting perfection. The exercise demonstrates how strength and conscious movement seamlessly integrate into the Pilates journey as the arms rise and fall against the wall supporting surface. In Pilates, Wall Angels inspire practitioners to go on a dynamic exploratory voyage that shapes a harmonious connection between body and soul.

4.4: Standing Wall Bicep Curls

Standing Wall Bicep Curls is a sophisticated workout from Wall Pilates that shows you how to shape arm power precisely and gracefully. Based on Pilates principles, this exercise targets the biceps, or the muscles at the front of the arms, by combining controlled motions with the wall's supporting surface. Let's examine the details of Standing Wall Bicep Curls and see how they work the biceps, improve the definition of the arms, and help create a balanced relationship between strength and fluidity of movement in the Pilates model.

1. Initial Position:

Start Building a Standing Wall To do bicep curls, place your back against the wall and ensure your head and tailbone are in touch with the wall across your whole spine. Place your feet a few inches from the wall and hip-width apart. Grasp little hand weights or apply resistance to your body. With your backs against the wall and your palms facing front, begin by completely extending your arms along the sides of your body. This first posture lays the groundwork for the subsequent deliberate motions, enabling the wall to provide encouraging direction.

2. Core Engagement and Alignment:

When doing Standing Wall Bicep Curls, ensure your spine stays in touch with the wall the whole time to maintain good alignment. Establish a solid base using your core muscles, especially your transverse abdominis. The alignment and core engagement promote regulated movement and minimize needless lower back strain. This basic configuration is essential to maximize the exercise's efficacy.

3. Regulated Bicep Curl Exercises:

The deliberate arm motions that imitate the traditional bicep curl action make Standing Wall Bicep Curls so effective. Breathe out and bend your elbows to bring your hands closer to your shoulders while keeping your back against the wall and the backs of your hands contacting it. When you lift weights or move your hands, concentrate on using your biceps, the muscles at the front of your arms. Take a breath and maintain the regulated speed as you stretch your arms back to the beginning position. This deliberate action engages The targeted muscle area mindfully and precisely.

4. Variations and Dynamic Movement:

Experiment with different versions to discover dynamic movement in standing wall bicep curls. To get the biceps working, add pulses at the top of the curl. Changing how your hands are positioned, such as turning your palms in the air as you lift, may be flexible, accommodating varying degrees of fitness and enabling more complex tasks. Because of the wall support's flexibility, you may try out various ranges of motion.

5. Breathing in Time with Movement:

When doing Standing Wall Bicep Curls, breath becomes your guide. As you start the curl, take a deep breath that expands your rib cage. As you raise the weights or move your hands, release all your air, contracting your core and concentrating on the deliberate movement. The coordinated breathing strengthens awareness and maintains the movement's smoothness. It is a rhythmic guide, encouraging control and elegance in the activity.

6. Stabilizing Wall Support:

The wall stabilizes the upper body during Standing Wall Bicep Curls. The backs of your hands and your whole spine continue to be in touch with the wall, acting as a constant anchor for stability. This supporting component benefits those trying to strengthen their arms or who may have wrist problems. With the wall support providing stability, practitioners can concentrate on honing their moves without worrying about losing their balance.

7. Conscious Attention to Biceps:

During standing wall bicep curls, focus on engaging your biceps. As the muscles at the front of the arms cooperate to regulate the curling action, you will feel their activation. By improving the mind-muscle connection, this conscious awareness makes it possible to explore bicep muscle activation more deliberately and subtly.

8. Alignment Verification and Adjustment:

Make sure your whole spine stays in touch with the wall by periodically checking your alignment while doing Standing Wall Bicep Curls. Adjustments may be made to suit varying fitness levels by changing the weight or the range of motion. The focus is on keeping the correct form to optimize the benefits of the exercise and reduce the chance of strain.

9. Building Arm Strength:

Biceps are worked out and strengthened by standing wall bicep curls. The deliberate motions provide more definition in the muscles at the front of the arms by enabling a sculpting investigation of bicep strength.

10. A Classy Resolution and Comeback:

Finally, lowering the weights or returning your hands to the beginning position is necessary for standing wall bicep curls. Breathe deeply, letting go of the biceps' contraction, and stand erect with purpose. The recovery phase is a crucial element that highlights the significance of deliberate recovery and the dynamic challenge. This thoughtful ending enhances the exercise's overall coherence and efficacy.

Advantages of Bicep Curls on the Wall:

1. **Development of Arm Strength**: Standing Wall Bicep Curls work the biceps and target them, which helps build arm strength.

2. **Controlled Movement:** This workout focuses on deliberate and precise arm motions that activate the targeted biceps.

3. **Breath-Movement Synchronization:** Bringing awareness and the exercise's fluidity together, synchronized breath and movement contribute to a mindful Pilates practice.

4. **Stabilizing Wall Support:** The wall is a stabilizing force, supporting confident and controlled execution. This is especially helpful for those who are trying to strengthen their arms.

5. **Mind-Body Connection:** Paying attention to how the bicep muscles contract with awareness strengthens the mind-body connection and promotes control and elegance in the activity.

6. **Adaptable for Varying Fitness Levels:** Standing Wall Bicep Curls are flexible, allowing adjustments to suit varying fitness levels and space for increasing difficulties.

7. **Posture Emphasis:** The exercise focuses on keeping the body in the correct posture, encouraging the best possible muscle activation, and avoiding needless lower back strain.

8. **Basis for Arm Awareness:** Standing Wall Bicep Curls is an essential exercise that develops bicep strength and awareness, laying the groundwork for further advancement in Pilates practice.

Wall Pilates's elegant choreography showcases Standing Wall Bicep Curls as a composed exercise, a lovely dance of

Controlled power, attentive participation, and accurate assistance. The exercise showcases the smooth combination of strength and thoughtful movement seen in the Pilates method as the arms raise and descend against the wall supporting surface. In Pilates, standing wall bicep curls allow practitioners to go on a dynamic exploratory voyage that shapes a harmonious relationship between body and soul.

4.5: High Plank with Shoulder Taps

A dynamic exercise from the Wall Pilates repertoire, the High Plank with Shoulder Taps reveals the secret to precise mastery of upper body control and core stability. This exercise, which has its roots in Pilates principles, skillfully combines the strength-enhancement elements of a high plank with the extra difficulty of shoulder taps, all while being stabilized by the wall. Let's explore the nuances of the High Plank with Shoulder Taps and how it develops upper body control, strengthens the core, and creates a harmonic relationship between strength and conscious movement in the context of the Pilates paradigm.

1. Initial Position:

Faced towards the wall, place your hands shoulder-height on the wall to begin the High Plank with Shoulder Taps. Stretch your legs out in a straight line from your head to your heels behind you. Place the feet hip-width apart. Make sure your spine remains neutral using your core muscles, and keep your hands planted on the wall. Starting from this stance lays the groundwork for the subsequent regulated movements, which use the wall for support and stability.

2. Core Engagement and Alignment:

Ensure your head and heels are straight to maintain good alignment throughout the High Plank with Shoulder Taps. Establish a solid base using your core muscles, especially your transverse abdominis. The alignment and core engagement promote regulated movement and minimize needless lower back strain. This basic configuration is essential to maximize the exercise's efficacy.

3. Managed Upper Plank Location:

With your body straight, stretch your arms to assume a high plank posture. You may concentrate on using your core muscles and maintaining perfect form by using the wall as a stabilizing support. The following dynamic shoulder taps are created on the controlled high plank posture.

4. Dynamic Shoulder Taps:

Tapping one hand at a time to the opposing shoulder makes the High Plank with Shoulder Taps so effective. Raise one hand off the wall while in the high plank position, then touch the shoulder of the other person. Repeat on the opposite side after returning the hand to the wall. The shoulder taps' dynamic aspect adds difficulty to the workout, necessitating more upper-body control and core stability. The wall makes precise and controlled motions possible, offering a continuous reference point.

5. Breathing in Time with Movement:

With Shoulder Taps, breath becomes an essential component of the High Plank. As you prepare for the shoulder tap, take a deep breath and stay in the high plank posture. Breathe completely as you raise one hand to touch the shoulder on the other side, utilizing your core muscles and paying attention to the deliberate action. Coordinated breathing contributes to a mindful Pilates practice by raising awareness and maintaining the exercise's flow.

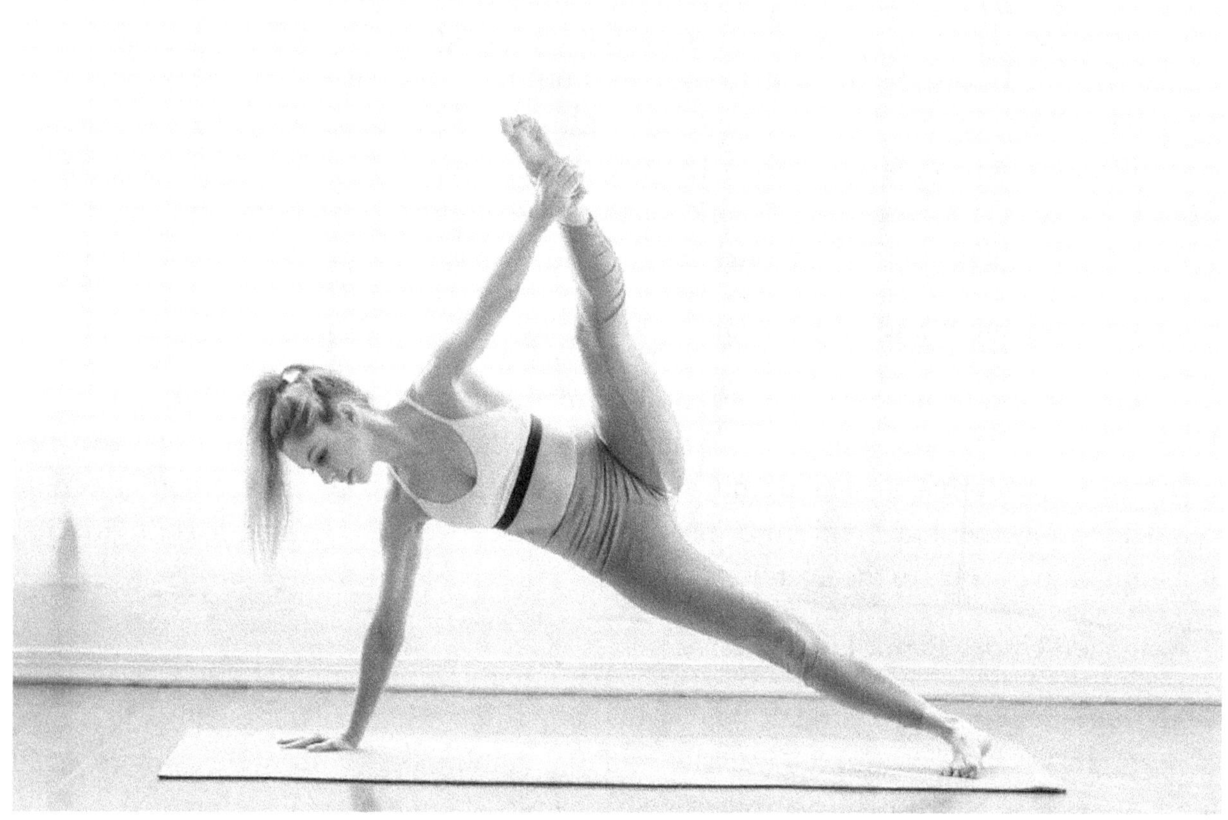

6. Supporting Stabilizing Wall:

The wall stabilizes the upper body during High Plank with Shoulder Taps. The hands continue to be in touch with the wall, acting as a constant source of support. This supporting component benefits those developing their upper body control and core strength. Thanks to the wall support's stabilizing effect, practitioners don't have to worry about losing their balance while honing their shoulder taps,

7. Consciously Maintaining Core Engagement:

Maintain focus on your core muscles throughout the High Plank with Shoulder Taps. During the dynamic shoulder taps, notice how your abs work to keep your body stable. By improving the mind-muscle link, this cognitive awareness makes it possible to explore core strength more deliberately and subtly.

8. Alignment Verification and Adjustment:

Make sure your alignment from head to heels is straight by periodically checking it throughout the High Plank with Shoulder Taps. Adjustments may be made to the shoulder taps' tempo or distance from the wall to suit varying degrees of fitness. The focus is on keeping the correct form to optimize the benefits of the exercise and reduce the chance of strain.

9. Development of Core Stability and Strength:

The High Plank with Shoulder Taps actively engages core stability and strength. The dynamic shoulder taps strengthen and regulate the abdominal area by testing the muscles that support the core.

10. A Classy Resolution and Comeback:

Returning to the beginning position with both hands on the wall is the last step in the High Plank with Shoulder Taps exercise. Take a deep breath, letting go of the contraction in your core, and purposefully stand up straight. The recovery phase is a crucial element that highlights the significance of deliberate recuperation and the dynamic challenge. This thoughtful ending enhances the exercise's overall coherence and efficacy.

High Plank with Shoulder Taps Benefits:

1. **Core Strength and Stability:** The abs are worked hard during the High Plank with Shoulder Taps, which actively activates and strengthens the core.

2. **Controlled High Plank posture:** This exercise strongly emphasizes a controlled high plank posture that encourages core muscular activation and accuracy.

3. **Breath-Movement Synchronization:** Bringing awareness and the exercise's fluidity together, synchronized breath and movement contribute to a mindful Pilates practice.

4. **Stabilizing Wall Support:** The wall is a stabilizing force, supporting confident and controlled execution. This is especially helpful for those who are trying to strengthen their core.

5. **Mind-Body Connection:** A deliberate emphasis on using the core muscles strengthens the mind-body connection and promotes control and elegance.

6. **Adaptable for Varied Fitness Levels**: The High Plank with Shoulder Taps is versatile, accommodating adaptations to suit varying fitness levels and offering space for more complex tasks.

7. **Posture Emphasis:** The exercise focuses on keeping the body in the correct posture, encouraging the best possible muscle activation, and avoiding needless lower back strain.

8. **Improving Upper Body Control:** The dynamic shoulder taps improve upper body control, which helps to build more muscular, more stable arms and shoulders.

9. **Basis for Core Awareness:** The High Plank combined with Shoulder Taps is an exercise that develops awareness and strength in the core muscles, laying the groundwork for more

Advancement in Pilates.

High Plank with Shoulder Taps is a dynamic exercise that combines strength, conscious engagement, and supporting accuracy seamlessly in Wall Pilates' elegant choreography. The exercise showcases the sleek fusion of upper body control and core strength in Pilates as the hands tap shoulders on the wall's supporting background. In the domain of Pilates, High Plank with Shoulder Taps encourages practitioners to go on a dynamic exploratory voyage that shapes a harmonious connection between body and soul.

4.6: Chest Stretch against Wall

A calm exercise in the Wall Pilates repertoire, Chest Stretch Against Wall reveals the subtle technique of opening and releasing tension. Based on Pilates principles, this exercise targets the front of the shoulders and the chest muscles by skillfully combining a light stretch with wall support. Let's examine the details of the Chest Stretch Against Wall and see how, in the context of the Pilates paradigm, it facilitates body-mind harmony, increases flexibility, and encourages relaxation.

1. Initial Position:

Start the Chest Stretch Against the Wall by facing the wall while standing a little distance away. Make sure both of your feet are firmly planted and hip-width apart. Place your hands slightly wider than shoulder-width apart on the wall at the shoulder. The palms of the arms should contact the wall, and the arms should be straight. With the wall providing stability and support, this beginning posture lays the groundwork for the subsequent moderate stretch.

2. Positioning and Conscious Posture:

When doing the Chest Stretch Against the Wall, ensure your shoulders are relaxed and your spine is straight. To establish stability, ground your feet and tighten your core for a solid base. To feel the stretch and relieve shoulder and chest tension, you must practice attentive posture and alignment, which cultivates awareness.

3. Soft Leaning Forward:

Lean your body softly so your chest touches the wall to begin the stretch. As you maintain your arms straight, concentrate on experiencing a little stretch over your chest and across your front shoulders. The controlled forward lean makes a progressive chest expansion possible, increasing flexibility and relieving tension in the upper body.

4. Controlled Breathing:

In the Chest, Stretch Against the Wall; breath acts as a compass. Breathe deeply to extend the rib cage and begin the forward lean. Breathe out completely as you ease into the pose, paying attention to let go of any tension in your shoulders and chest. Breath and movement in unison improves awareness, which helps the exercise flow and fosters a mindful Pilates practice.

5. Supporting the Wall and Unwinding:

You may surrender into the stretch during the Chest Stretch Against The Wall since the wall provides soft support for your hands and arms. The hands maintain contact with the wall, always offering a stable reference point for all supporting components. It benefits those trying to improve their chest flexibility or want a little stretch.

6. Conscientious Chest Dilation:

During the stretch, pay close attention to how your chest expands. Sensate the front of the shoulders and the muscles in your chest growing slightly. The mind-muscle link is improved by this cognitive awareness, enabling a more complex and deliberate stretch experience.

7. Unwinding and Giving Up:

Encourage a sensation of relaxation and letting go as you sink into the pose. Let go of whatever stress you carry in your shoulders and chest, allowing the mild stretch to relax and energize these regions. ThoughtThe controlled forward lean creates a journey of relaxation that makes general well-being.

8. Alignment Verification and Adjustment:

During the Chest Stretch Against the Wall, periodically check your alignment to ensure your shoulders are relaxed and your spine is straight. Adjustments may be made to allow varying degrees of comfort by running the distance from the wall or the intensity of the stretch. The goal is to create a stretch that is restorative and revitalizing.

9. Improving Chest Flexibility:

The chest muscles are actively engaged, improving their flexibility with the Chest Stretch Against Wall. Over time, increasing flexibility is promoted by the regulated stretch supported by the wall and permits a progressive chest expansion.

10. A Classy Closure and Conscientious Departure:

The last stretch, Chest Stretch Against Wall, involves a gentle stand-up. Take a deep breath and notice how your chest expands. As you consciously stand up straight, acknowledge the increased opening in your shoulders and chest. The exercise is more fluid and effective overall when the elegant release from the stretch is executed.

Advantages of Wall-Based Chest Stretches:

1. **Chest and Shoulder Release:** Leaning against the wall with your arms extended allows your chest and shoulders to release tension, which helps you relax.

2. **Gentle Stretch and Opening:** This exercise expands the chest to improve flexibility and space diversion.

3. ** Breath-Movement Synchronization:** This technique adds to a mindful Pilates exercise by enhancing awareness and sustaining the stretch's smoothness.

4. **Wall Support for Stability:** By acting as a supporting component, the wall makes the stretch more stable and guarantees a pleasant and regulated experience.

5. **Mindful Posture and Alignment:** Focusing on cautious posture and alignment lays the groundwork for a deliberate and more successful stretch that enhances well-being.

6. **Relaxation and Letting Go:** This practice helps practitioners let go of stress and enjoy a peaceful stretch by promoting relaxation and letting go.

7. **Adaptable for Varied Comfort Levels:** The Chest Stretch Against Wall is a mild stretch that can be modified to suit various comfort levels and may be calming for those seeking a more gentle workout.

8. **Enhanced Chest Flexibility:** The deliberate stretch supports general upper body mobility by improving the flexibility of the chest muscles.

9. **Mind-Body Connection:** Encouragement strengthens the mind-body connection and brings awareness of the feelings in the chest and shoulders throughout the stretch; the exegesis for Upper Body Awareness:** The fundamental exercise is a chest stretch against the wall.

Stretch that prepares the body for future advancement in Pilates practice by increasing awareness and flexibility in the shoulders and chest.

Chest Stretch Against Wall is a calming exercise that combines attentive involvement, supporting accuracy, and a delicate dance of release in Wall Pilates' elegant choreography. The practice becomes a monument to the exquisite fusion of flexibility and conscious movement within the Pilates journey as the chest expands and tension releases against the soothing wall. In the Pilates universe, Chest Stretch Against Wall enables practitioners to go on a peaceful exploratory voyage that shapes a harmonious connection between body and soul.

4.7: Wall-Assisted Arm Circles

One of the most sophisticated exercises in the Wall Pilates repertoire, Wall-Assisted Arm Circles creates a harmonious combination of stability and shoulder mobility. Based on Pilates principles, this exercise combines gentle arm circles seamlessly with the wall's supporting guidance. It targets the shoulders and improves upper body control. Let's get into the details of Wall-Assisted Arm Circles and see how this Pilates paradigm enhances shoulder mobility, increases stability, and creates a harmonic relationship between strength and conscious movement.

1. Initial Position:

With your side to the wall and ensuring your arm can easily reach the wall, begin Wall-Assisted Arm Circles. Place your feet hip-width apart and stand with your back to the wall. Place your palm at shoulder height against the wall with your fingers pointed upward. Starting from this stance creates a foundation for the smooth arm circles by using the wall as a guide for deliberate movement.

2. Core Engagement and Alignment:

Keep your body straight during Wall-Assisted Arm Circles to ensure optimal alignment. Establish a solid base using your core muscles, especially your transverse abdominis. The alignment and core engagement promote regulated movement and minimize needless lower back strain. This basic configuration is essential to maximize the exercise's efficacy.

3. Arm Circles with Control:

The regulated action of circling your arm is the foundation of Wall-Assisted Arm Circles. Start the circular motion by drawing little circles in clockwise and counterclockwise directions with your hand on the wall. The wall acts as a stabilizing reference, facilitating deliberate and accurate activation of the shoulder muscles. Keep your speed steady and fluid as you go around the circles.

4. Variations and Dynamic Movement:

Change the size and speed of the circles to investigate dynamic movement inside Wall-Assisted Arm Circles. As your shoulder muscles warm up, think about beginning with smaller circles and progressively increasing the diameter. Try rotating in both clockwise and counterclockwise directions to activate various muscle fibers. Because of the wall support's flexibility, you may modify the workout to suit your demands.

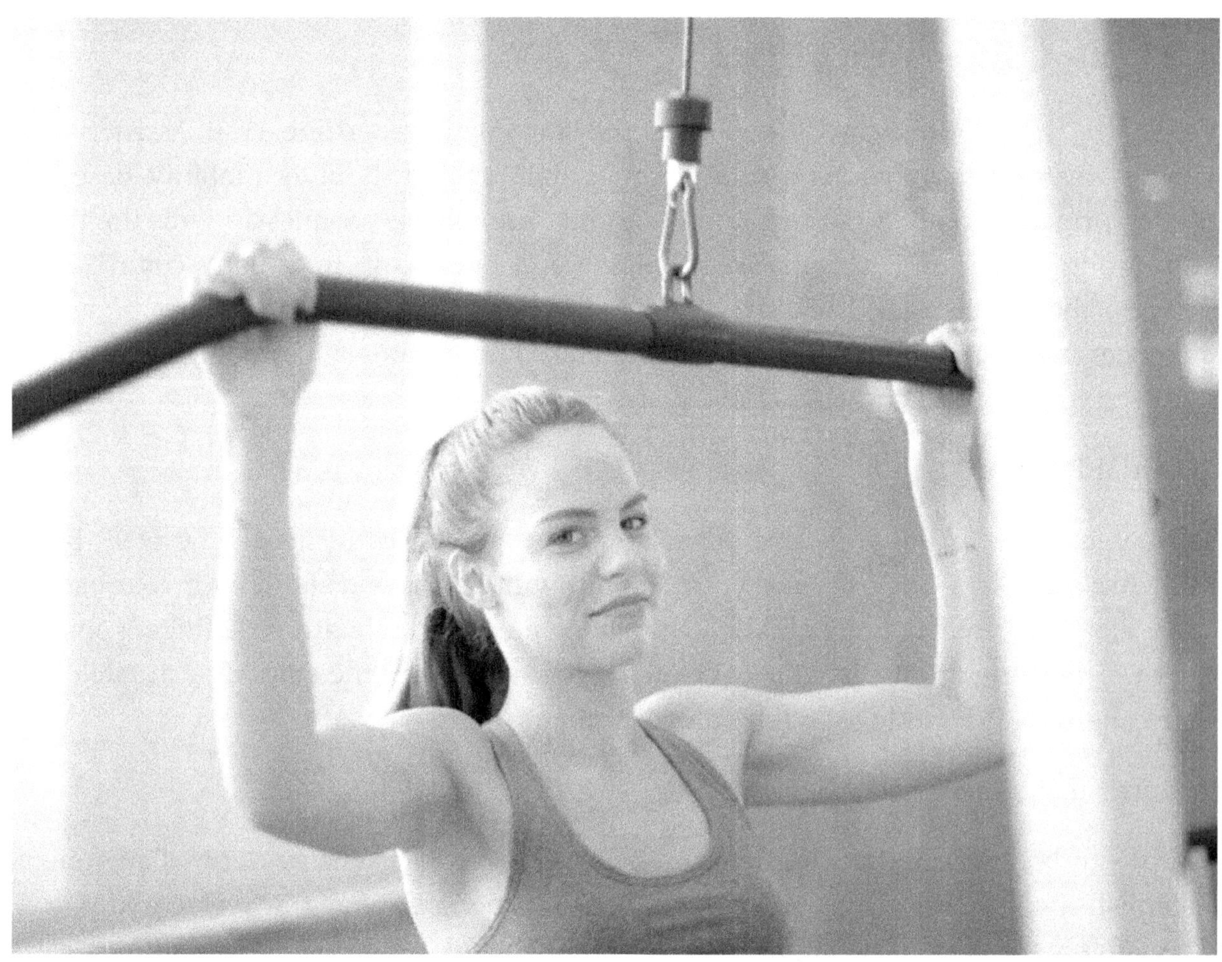

5. Breathing in Time with Movement:

When doing Wall-Assisted Arm Circles, breath becomes a guiding principle. As you draw the circles, take a deep breath that expands your rib cage. As you finish each turn, let out all of your breaths, utilizing your core muscles and your attention to the deliberate movement. The coordinated breathing strengthens awareness and maintains the movement's smoothness. It is a rhythmic guide, encouraging control and elegance in the activity.

6. Stabilizing Wall Support:

During Wall-Assisted Arm Circles, the arm in motion is stabilized by the wall. The hand maintains its touch with the wall, acting as a constant stabilizing anchor. Those who are recuperating from shoulder injuries or seeking to improve shoulder mobility may particularly benefit from this supporting component. Practitioners don't have to worry about losing their balance while honing their arm circles because of the wall support's stabilizing effect.

7. Paying Attention to Shoulder Muscles:

Keep your attention focused and mindfully on your shoulder muscles while you do wall-assisted arm circles. As these muscles cooperate to perform the circular motion, you may feel them become active. By improving the mind-muscle link, this cognitive awareness makes it possible to explore shoulder mobility more deliberately and subtly.

8. Alignment Verification and Adjustment:

During Wall-Assisted Arm Circles, periodically check your alignment to make sure your arm is comfortable and straight. Adjustments may be made to suit varying fitness levels by changing the pace or the size of the circles. To optimize the bench, the focus is on keeping the correct form toits of the exercise and reducing the chance of strain; the focus is on shoulder Mobility:**

9. Wall-Assisted Arm Circles:

These exercises actively involve and improve shoulder joint mobility. The regulated circular action fosters an Increased range of motion, which enables a beautiful exploration of shoulder mobility.

10. A Classy Resolution and Comeback:

Wall-assisted arm Circles end with a gentle arm descent that releases the tension in the shoulder muscles. Breathe deeply, appreciating your shoulders' increased range of motion, then rise straight and purposefully. The recovery phase is a crucial element that highlights the significance of deliberate recovery and the dynamic challenge. This thoughtful ending enhances the exercise's overall coherence and efficacy.

Wall-Assisted Arm Circle Benefits:

1. **Shoulder Mobility Enhancement:** By actively engaging and enhancing the shoulder joint's mobility, Wall-Assisted Arm Circles provide an expanded range of motion.

2. **Controlled Movement:** This exercise focuses on precise, deliberate activation of the shoulder muscles via controlled circular movements.

3. **Breath-Movement Synchronization:** Bringing awareness and the exercise's fluidity together, synchronized breath and movement contribute to a mindful Pilates practice.

4. **Stabilizing Wall Support:** The wall is a stabilizing force, supporting confident and controlled execution. This is especially helpful for those trying to improve their shoulder mobility.

5. **Mind-Body Connection:** Paying attention to activating the shoulder muscles mindfully strengthens the mind-body connection and promotes control and grace in the exercise.

6. **Adaptable for Varying Fitness Levels:** Wall-Assisted Arm Circles are flexible, allowing adjustments to suit varying fitness levels and space for increasing difficulties.

7. **Posture Emphasis:** The exercise focuses on keeping the body in the correct posture, encouraging the best possible muscle activation, and avoiding needless lower back strain.

8. **Dynamic Shoulder Warm-Up:** Wall-assisted arm Circles are a great way to warm up your shoulder muscles and prepare them for a Pilates class.

9. **Wall-Assisted Arm Circles:** The Basis for Shoulder Awareness Function as a fundamental exercise that increases shoulder joint awareness and mobility, laying the groundwork for further Pilates practice advancements.

10. 10. **Improving Upper Body Control:** The dynamic arm circles help to improve upper body control by strengthening and stabilizing the arms and shoulders.

Wall-assisted arm Circles become a dynamic movement in the elegant choreography of Wall Pilates, a symphony of mobility, attentive involvement, and supporting accuracy. The exercise showcases how the Pilates method integrates shoulder mobility and stability as the arm moves beautifully in circles against the wall supporting background. In Pilates, Wall-Assisted Arm Circles allow practitioners to go on a dynamic exploratory voyage that shapes a harmonious connection between body and soul.

Chapter 5: Spine and Posture Alignment

5.1: Wall Cat-Cow Stretch

Nestled within the Wall Pilates repertoire, the Wall Cat-Cow Stretch creates a smooth, flowing symphony of flexion and extension of the spine. Based on Pilates' fundamentals, this exercise skillfully combines the classic Cat-Cow stretch with the additional wall support. Within the Pilates paradigm, the Wall Cat-Cow Stretch is a vital exercise that respects the spine's natural range of motion, cultivates flexibility, and promotes a conscious connection between body and breath.

1. Initial Position:

With your back to the Wall and about an arm's length away, start the Wall Cat-Cow Stretch. Step with your feet hip-width apart to provide a sturdy base. Place your hands at shoulder height on the Wall with your fingers spread widely for best support. This first alignment creates a bond with the Wall, providing a stable background for the following smooth motions.

2. Core Engagement and Alignment:

When doing the Wall Cat-Cow Stretch, ensure your spine is in a neutral posture to maintain good alignment. To establish stability, contract the transverse abdominis and other core muscles. A balanced flow of spinal flexion and extension is made possible by alignment and core engagement, which also helps to avoid needless strain and encourage a regulated stretch.

3. Smooth Cat-Cow Motions:

The Wall's basic idea: The secret to the Cat-Cow Stretch is how smoothly the body moves against the Wall. Exhale, circle your back (the cat posture) and plant your hands firmly on the Wall to begin the stretch. Take a deep breath, arch your back, push your pelvis forward, and raise your head into the cow posture. The Wall is a comforting cue for the movement, facilitating a seamless change from the Cow to the Cat posture. Examine the spine's soft curvature, paying particular attention to each vertebra's articulation.

4. Breathing in Time with Movement:

Taking a breath becomes essential to doing the Wall Cat-Cow Stretch. Take a deep breath as you extend your chest and let your belly fall into the Cow posture. As you enter the Cat posture, release all your air, contracting your abdominal muscles and curving your spine. Inspiring a mindful Pilates practice and strengthening the link between breath and motion, the coordinated breath and movement improve awareness.

5. Wall Assistance for Managed Motion:

Throughout the Wall Cat-Cow Stretch, your hands are stabilized by the Wall. This support provides a feeling of stability that may be especially helpful for those working on their spine flexibility or those with balance issues. It enables regulated and precise movements. By acting as a stable anchor, the Wall helps practitioners concentrate on the quality of their movements.

6. Conscientious Attention to Spinal Articulation:

During the Wall Cat-Cow Stretch, consciously concentrate on the spine's articulation. As each vertebra travels via the undulating action, feel each one in turn. By improving the mind-muscle link, this cognitive awareness makes it possible to explore spinal flexion and extension more deliberately and subtly.

7. Awareness of the Tailbone and Pelvic Movement:

Pay attention to how your pelvis and tailbone move during the Wall Cat-Cow Stretch. Allow the pelvis to lean forward during the cat-to-cow transition to gently arch the lower back. To circle the spine and move the tailbone towards the floor, adopt the Cat posture by contracting your abdominal muscles. The stretch is more effective overall because of this little pelvic movement.

8. Alignment Verification and Adjustment:

Ensure your spine stays in a smooth motion and your hands are at shoulder height by periodically checking your alignment while doing the Wall Cat-Cow Stretch. To allow varying degrees of comfort, adjustments may be made by changing the distance from the Wall or the intensity of the stretch. The goal is to create a stretch that is both refreshing and invigorating.

9. Improvement of Spinal Flexibility:

Spinning flexibility is actively engaged and improved with the Wall Cat-Cow Stretch. Gradually, the regulated motions provide a delicate exploration of the whole range of motion of the spine, leading to improved flexibility. Thanks to the wall support, this investigation may take place in a secure and regulated setting.

10. A Classy Resolution and Comeback:

To release the Wall Cat-Cow Stretch, take a deep breath and stand back up in a neutral stance. As you consciously stand up straight, acknowledge the restored flexibility in your back. The recovery phase is a crucial element that highlights the significance of deliberate recovery and the dynamic challenge. This thoughtful ending enhances the exercise's overall coherence and efficacy.

Wall Cat-Cow Stretch Benefits:

1. **Spinal Flexibility Enhancement:** The Wall Cat-Cow Stretch gently explores the whole range of motion of the spine by actively engaging and enhancing spinal flexibility.

2. **Controlled Cat-Cow Movements:** This exercise focuses on smooth, wall-mounted Cat-Cow motions that encourage agility and conscious back activation.

3. **Breath-Movement Synchronization:** This technique adds to a mindful Pilates exercise by enhancing awareness and sustaining the stretch's smoothness.

4. **Stabilizing Wall Support:** The Wall acts as a stabilizing force, supporting confident and controlled execution—especially helpful for those focusing on improving spinal flexibility.

5. **Mind-Body link:** A deliberate concentration on spinal articulation strengthens the link between mind and body, promoting control and elegance.

6. **Flexible for Varied Comfort Levels:** The Wall Cat-Cow Stretch is a calming stretch for practitioners of all skill levels and is flexible enough to adjust to varying comfort levels.

7. **Posture Emphasis:** The exercise emphasizes keeping the spine in the ideal posture, encouraging maximum spinal engagement, and avoiding needless lower back strain.

8. **Pelvic Movement Awareness:** This stretch helps to create a more conscious and deliberate sense of spinal flexion and extension by improving awareness of pelvic movement and tailbone posture.

9. **Gentle Release of Tension:** The Wall Cat-Cow Stretch's wavy motion facilitates a mild release of spinal tension, fostering suppleness and relaxation.

10. **Basis for Spinal Health:** The Wall Cat-Cow Stretch is an essential exercise that develops spinal awareness, flexibility, and health. It lays the groundwork for more advanced Pilates exercises.

The Wall Cat-Cow Stretch is a revitalizing exercise that appears in the elegant choreography of Wall Pilates. It is a fluid waltz of spinal flexion and extension, attentive involvement, and supporting accuracy. The exercise serves as a testimony to the seamless integration of flexibility and conscious movement within the Pilates journey, as the spine smoothly undulates against the comfortable Wall. In Pilates, the Wall Cat-Cow Stretch enables practitioners to go on a voyage of fluid exploration, creating a harmonic connection between body and soul.

5.2: Standing Chest Opener

Nestled in the Wall Pilates world, the Standing Chest Opener is a revolutionary exercise that improves posture and heart-centric flexibility. This exercise, which has its roots in Pilates fundamentals, skillfully combines the wall's supporting embrace with the elegance of an open chest. In the Pilates paradigm, the Standing Chest Opener becomes a ritual of expansion, promoting flexibility, releasing tension, and a conscious connection between body and breath.

1. Initial Position:

Starting at a comfortable distance, face the wall with your back while doing the Standing Chest Opener. Plant your feet hip-width apart to provide a firm base. Reach back and put your hands shoulder-height on the wall with your fingers pointing down. With the wall supporting the following chest-opening action, this beginning posture lays the groundwork for the transforming stretch.

2. Core Engagement and Alignment:

Ensure your spine is in a neutral posture to do the Standing Chest Opener with good alignment. To establish stability, contract the transverse abdominis and other core muscles. To facilitate a harmonic stretch and avoid needless strain, the alignment and core engagement create the scene for a regulated release of tension in the shoulders and chest.

3. Arm Extension Under Control:

The deliberate extension of your arms behind you makes the Standing Chest Opener so effective. Pay attention to the arms' extension as you push your hands against the wall. Lift the gaze to the ceiling and let the chest open naturally. A steady support from the wall allows for a slow, deliberate movement. As the chest opens, investigate the sense of expansion and release.

4. Breathing in Time with Movement:

In the Standing Chest Opener, breathing becomes essential. Breathe deeply while you open your chest, spread your arms, and widen your rib cage. To engage the core muscles and provide a more profound release in the shoulders and chest, completely exhale while you hold the stretch. Breath and movement in unison improve awareness, cultivating a mindful Pilates practice and strengthening the link between breath and the expansive stretch.

5. Controlled Release Wall Support:

The wall provides stable guidance for gradual release during the Standing Chest Opener. The hands continue to be in touch with the wall, acting as a constant source of support. Thanks to this support, the upper back, shoulders, and chest may gradually relax. By taking on a nurturing role, the wall helps practitioners concentrate on the quality of the stretch.

6. Concise Attention to Chest Expansion:

During the Standing Chest Opener, direct your focused attention to the expansion of your chest. Feel the collarbones widening and the muscles in the chest opening up. By improving the mind-muscle link, this cognitive awareness makes it possible to feel chest flexibility more deliberately and subtly.

7. Knowledge of Shoulder Blades:

During the Standing Chest Opener, pay close attention to how your shoulder blades move and are positioned. As your chest expands, let the shoulder blades slowly down your back to facilitate a wide-open, comfortable release. The stretch is more effective overall because of its focus on shoulder blade mobility.

8. Alignment Verification and Adjustment:

Throughout the Standing Chest Opener, periodically check your alignment to ensure your spine is neutral and your hands are at shoulder height. Adjustments may be made to allow varying degrees of comfort by running the distance from the wall or the intensity of the stretch. The goal is to create a stretch that is both energizing and spacious.

9. Improving Chest Flexibility:

Chest flexibility is actively engaged and improved with the Standing Chest Opener. With time, more flexibility is encouraged by the smooth exploration of the chest's whole range of motion, made possible by the wall-supported, controlled extension of the arms.

Thanks to the wall support, this investigation may take place in a secure and regulated setting.

10. A Classy Resolution and Comeback:

The Standing Chest Opener concludes with a gentle release of the stretch and a deep breath to recognize the expanding feeling in the chest. Take a purposeful stance and enjoy your newfound transparency. The recovery phase is a crucial element that highlights the significance of deliberate recovery and the dynamic challenge. This thoughtful ending enhances the exercise's overall coherence and efficacy.

A Standing Chest Opener's Benefits

1. **Enhancing Chest Flexibility**: The Standing Chest Opener actively engages and improves chest flexibility, making it easy to explore the chest's whole range of motion with elegance.

2. **Controlled Arm Extension:** This exercise focuses on a deliberate and precise extension of the arms, engaging the chest muscles with awareness.

3. **Breath-Movement Synchronization:** This technique adds to a mindful Pilates exercise by enhancing awareness and sustaining the stretch's smoothness.

4. **Stabilizing Wall Support**: The wall stabilizes, supporting confident and controlled execution. This is especially helpful for those who are practicing chest flexibility.

5. **Mind-Body Connection:** Chest expansion is a mindful concentration that strengthens the mind-body connection.

We are Encouraging control and elegance throughout the workout.

1. **Adaptable for Varied Comfort Levels**: The Standing Chest Opener is flexible, adjusting varying degrees of comfort and space for progressively more complex tasks.

2. **Posture Emphasis:** The exercise emphasizes keeping the body in the correct posture, encouraging chest engagement, and avoiding needless shoulder strain.

3. **Shoulder Blade Awareness:** The stretch encourages awareness of the movement of the shoulder blades, which helps to make the feeling of expanding the chest more subtle and deliberate.

4. **Gentle Release of Tension:** By carefully extending the arms against the wall, you may gently release the tension in your chest, which helps you feel more at ease and roomy.

5. **Basis for Heart-Centric Posture:** The Standing Chest Opener is an exercise that increases awareness, flexibility, and posture around the heart. It also lays the groundwork for more advanced Pilates poses.

The Standing Chest Opener is a transforming exercise that combines attentive involvement, supporting accuracy, and seamless chest flexibility. It is best seen in the elegant choreography of Wall Pilates. The practice showcases how openness and thoughtful movement seamlessly integrate into the Pilates journey as the chest opens gently against the soothing wall. In Pilates, Standing Chest Opener encourages practitioners to explore an expanded exploratory voyage that shapes a harmonious connection between body and soul.

5.3: Wall-Assisted Forward Bend

The Wall-Assisted Forward Bend is a beautiful way to release tension and invite more flexibility. It is an excellent addition to the Wall Pilates repertory. Based on the basic principles of Pilates, this exercise combines the classic forward bend with the wall for increased support. Within the Pilates paradigm, the Wall-Assisted Forward Bend becomes a healing ritual supporting the conscious release, the spine's suppleness, and a deep connection between body and breath.

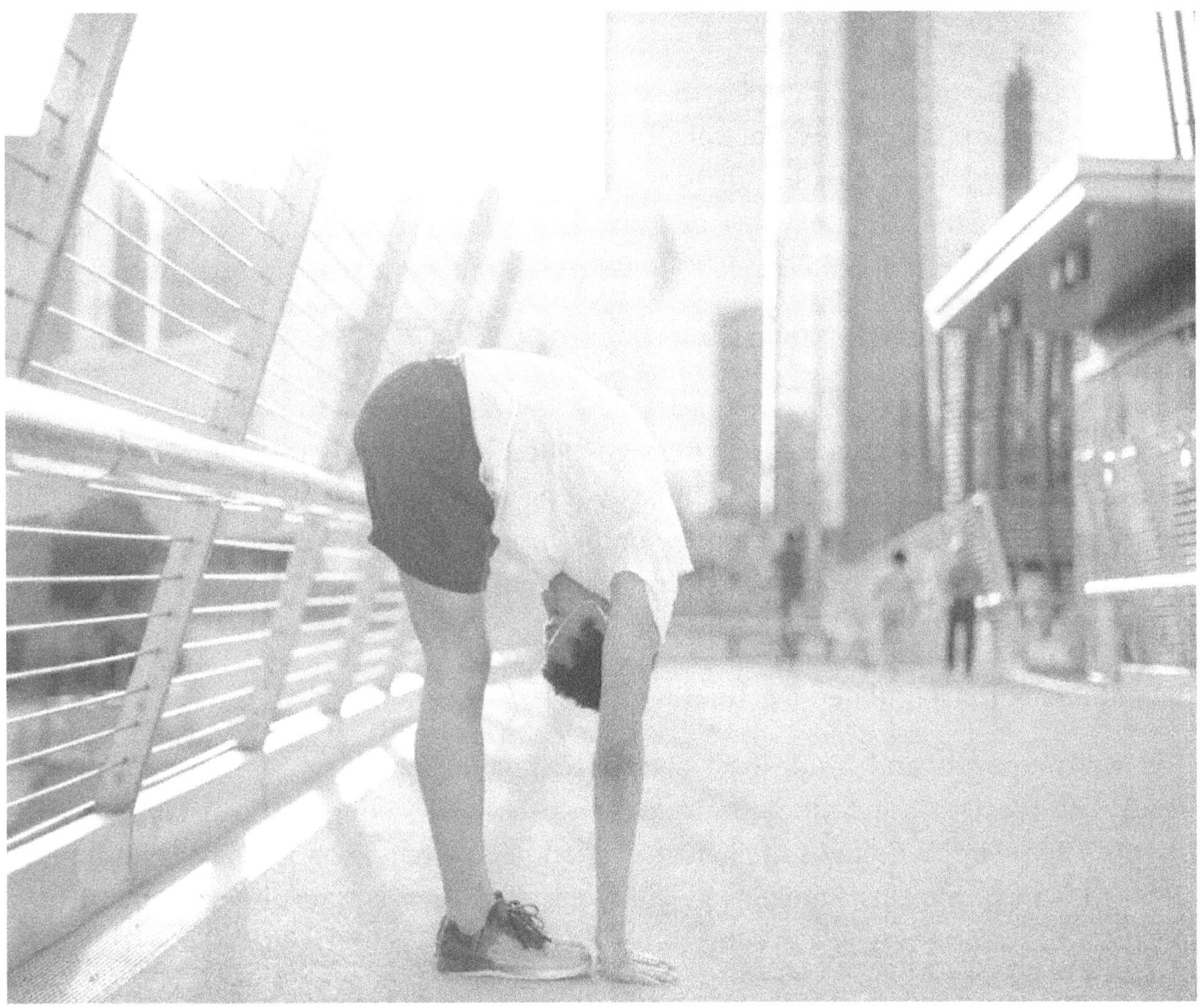

1. Initial Position:

Standing with your back against the wall and your feet hip-width apart, begin the Wall-Assisted Forward Bend. To make a connection, let your tailbone softly touch against the wall. Raise your arms and rest your palms and fingers on the wall. By beginning here, you establish a basic alignment and use the wall as a support structure for the next forward bend.

2. Core Engagement and Alignment:

When doing the Wall-Assisted Forward Bend, ensure your spine is in a neutral posture to maintain good alignment. To establish stability, contract your core muscles, especially your transverse abdominis. In addition to avoiding needless strain and encouraging a controlled release of tension in the spine, alignment and core engagement prepare the body for a harmonic forward bend.

3. Regulated Forward Extension:

The controlled bending of the spine makes the Wall-Assisted Forward Bend so effective. Let your upper body collapse forward by inhaling and pivoting at the hips to start the exercise. Your hands maintain pressure on the wall, acting as a solid anchor. The wall support guides the action, which guarantees a slow and deliberate forward flexion. Bend forward and explore how it feels to have the spine unfurl and release tension.

4. Breathing in Time with Movement:

Breath becomes an essential component of the Forward Bend with Wall Assistance. Take a deep breath and raise your arms over your head to get ready to bend. As you begin the forward bend, release all your air, activating your core muscles and enabling your upper body to fold. Breath and movement in unison improve awareness, cultivating a mindful Pilates practice and strengthening the link between breath and the unfolding stretch.

5. Wall Assist for Regulated Decline:

The wall supports and guides the controlled fall during the Wall-Assisted Forward Bend. The hands continue to be in touch with the wall, acting as a constant source of support. This support allows the hamstrings and spine to relax gradually, resulting in a deliberate and controlled movement. The wall takes on a comforting aura that draws practitioners in and helps them concentrate on the quality of the stretch.

6. Pay Close Attention to Spinal Flexibility:

Pay close attention to your spine's flexibility while you do the Wall-Assisted Forward Bend. Sensation feels each vertebra as it flexes forward one after the other, releasing tension gradually. By improving the mind-muscle link, this conscious awareness makes it possible to experience spinal flexion in a more complex and deliberate way.

7. Stretching the Hamstrings and Hip Hinge:

The Wall-Assisted Forward Bend is predominantly a hip-based technique; therefore, pay attention to the hip hinge. The hamstrings may be specifically stretched with this deliberate hip hinge. While keeping the forward bend, notice how your legs are becoming longer. The whole stretch has more depth when combined with the hamstring and hip hinge.

8. Alignment Verification and Adjustment:

Check your alignment often while doing the Wall-Assisted Forward Bend to ensure your spine is neutral and your hands are at shoulder height. Adjustments may be made to allow varying degrees of comfort by running the distance from the wall or the intensity of the stretch. The goal is to create a stretch that is both refreshing and invigorating.

9. Relaxation and Spinal Release:

The Forward, Aided by the Wall Bend, actively releases spinal tension. Feel the vertebrae gently lengthening and the spine decompressing as you bend forward. The deliberate descent enhances a therapeutic experience by fostering a feeling of relaxation and flexibility in the back.

10. A Classy Resolution and Comeback:

Finalizing the Forward-Assisted Wall Bend is gradually returning to an upright posture while taking a deep breath to recognize the space in the spine. Take a purposeful stance and enjoy the fresh freedom. The recovery phase is a crucial element that highlights the significance of deliberate recovery and the dynamic challenge. This thoughtful ending enhances the exercise's overall coherence and efficacy.

Wall-Assisted Forward Bend Benefits:

1. **Spinal Flexibility Enhancement:** The Wall-Assisted Forward Bend facilitates a controlled release of spinal tension by actively engaging and improving spinal flexibility.

2. **Controlled Forward Flexion**: This exercise promotes accuracy and deliberate activation of the back muscles by emphasizing controlled flexion of the spine.

3. **Breath-Movement Synchronization:** This technique adds to a mindful Pilates exercise by enhancing awareness and sustaining the stretch's smoothness.

4. **Stabilizing Wall Support:** The wall acts as a stabilizing force, supporting confident and controlled execution—especially helpful for those focusing on improving spinal flexibility.

5. **Mind-Body link:** A deliberate attention to spinal flexibility strengthens the link between mind and body, promoting control and elegance.

6. **Adaptable for Varying Comfort Levels:** The Wall-Assisted Forward Bend is flexible, enabling adjustments to suit various.

Comfort zones and making space forever more complex tasks.

1. **Hip Hinge and Hamstring Stretch**: This deliberate hip hinge focuses on the hamstring stretch, deepening the total stretch and increasing the back of the legs' flexibility.

2. **Alignment stress:** The exercise stresses keeping the back muscles engaged optimally, avoiding needless effort, and maintaining correct alignment.

3. **Gentle Release of Tension:** The deliberate lowering against the wall permits a mild release of spinal tension, encouraging flexibility and relaxation.

4. **Basis for Spinal Health:** The Wall-Assisted Forward Bend is an essential Pilates exercise that develops spinal awareness, flexibility, and health. It also lays the groundwork for more advanced Pilates techniques.

The Wall-Assisted Forward Bend, in the elegant choreography of Wall Pilates, is a delicate unfurling, a fluid waltz of spinal flexibility, conscious release, and supporting accuracy. The practice becomes a testimony to the seamless integration of controlled movement and mindful stretch within the Pilates journey as the spine softly bends forward against the soothing background of the wall. Wall-Assisted Forward Bend is a Pilates exercise that encourages practitioners to harmoniously explore their bodies and spirits while traveling on a therapeutic trip.

5.4: Pelvic Clock

One of the most complex movements in the Wall Pilates repertoire is the Pelvic Clock, which creates a beautiful dance between pelvic mobility and core stability. Based on Pilates's fundamentals, this exercise integrates the finer points of pelvic articulation with the wall's supporting canvas. Within the Pilates paradigm, the Pelvic Clock emerges as a transforming ritual that fosters a deep connection between body and breath, enhances pelvic flexibility, and cultivates conscious awareness.

1. Initial Position:

Standing with your back to the wall and maintaining a neutral spine and a comfortable distance from the wall are the first steps in executing the Pelvic Clock. Step with your feet hip-width apart to provide a firm base. You may rest your arms at your sides or place your hands on your hips. This initial posture creates the supporting base for the following complex motions.

2. Core Engagement and Alignment:

When doing the Pelvic Clock, ensure your core muscles—particularly the transverse abdominis—are contracted and your spine is neutral. By avoiding needless strain and encouraging a deliberate study of pelvic articulation, the alignment and core engagement provide a secure foundation for the subtle pelvic motions.

3. Motions of Pelvic Articulation:

The complex articulation of the pelvis via a sequence of motions mimicking a clock's face is the fundamental component of the Pelvic Clock. Move your pelvis in the following controlled directions: forward, backwards, side-to-side, and circular. Imagine your pelvis as the center of the clock. The wall acts as a stable background, directing and bolstering the accuracy of pelvic articulation. Experiment with the range of motion while keeping your grip on the wall steady.

4. Breathing in Time with Movement:

Breath becomes a vital part of the Pelvic Clock. As you prepare for the pelvic movement, take a deep breath and let your rib cage stretch. Completely release your breath while you contract your abdominal muscles and move your pelvis in the desired direction. Breath and movement synchronization improves awareness, which promotes mindful Pilates practice and strengthens the link between breath and subtle pelvic articulation.

5. Wall Assistance for Managed Motion:

The wall of the Pelvic Clock provides stability and guidance for deliberate movement—the continuous attachment to the wall allows for a fluid and deliberate investigation of the pelvic clock movements. By acting as a stabilizing force, the wall helps practitioners concentrate on the accuracy and caliber of pelvic articulation.

6. Pelvic Awareness with a Mindful Focus:

During the Pelvic Clock, pay close attention to your pelvic awareness. Explore the clock movements and experience the minute revolutions and shifts. By improving the mind-muscle link, this cognitive awareness makes pelvic motion more subtle and deliberate.

7. Examining Clock Directions:

Start your investigation by shifting your pelvis in the different clockwise directions. Perform tilts in all directions, including forward, backward, side-to-side, and circular movements. Every orientation enhances the pelvis' total range of motion and flexibility, which helps the pelvic area feel more liberated.

8. Alignment Verification and Adjustment:

Ensure your pelvis articulates smoothly, and your spine stays neutral by periodically checking your alignment while doing the Pelvic Clock. Adjustments may be performed to accommodate varying degrees of comfort by changing the distance from the wall or the strength of the motions. The goal is to explore the pelvic clock in a controlled and flexible manner.

9. Core Connection and Pelvic Stability:

The Pelvic Clock is a unique combination of core stability and pelvic mobility. The core muscles must be used throughout the regulated motions to support and stabilize the pelvis. The combination of core stability and pelvic mobility generally enhances functional strength and balance.

10. A Classy Resolution and Comeback:

Returning to a neutral standing posture and taking a deep breath to recognize the subtle changes in pelvic awareness are the last steps in completing the Pelvic Clock. Take a purposeful stance and acknowledge your newfound connection. The recovery phase is a crucial element that highlights the significance of deliberate recovery and the dynamic challenge. This thoughtful ending enhances the exercise's overall coherence and efficacy.

11. Pelvic Mobility Enhancement:

The Pelvic Clock actively promotes pelvic mobility, enabling a controlled exploration of pelvic articulation in different directions. This is one of the Pelvic Clock's benefits.

1. **Core Stability Fusion:** This exercise creates a harmonic link between the pelvic area and the core muscles by smoothly fusing core stability with pelvic mobility.

2. Breath-Movement Synchronization: This technique adds to a mindful Pilates exercise by promoting awareness and maintaining the pelvic clock's fluidity.

3. **Stabilizing Wall Support:** Especially helpful for those working on pelvic mobility, the wall acts as a stabilizing force, offering support for a controlled and confident execution.

4. **Mind-Body link:** A deliberate emphasis on pelvic awareness strengthens the link between mind and body, promoting control and elegance.

5. **Adaptable for Varied Comfort Levels:** The Pelvic Clock is flexible, allowing for adjustments to suit varying comfort levels and opportunities for increasing difficulties.

6. **Clock Directions Exploration**: This exercise encourages practitioners to investigate several clock directions, which leads to a complete and freeing sensation of pelvic mobility.

7. **Alignment focus:** The Pelvic Clock focuses on keeping the body in the proper alignment, encouraging optimum core muscle activation and reducing needless strain.

8. **Nuanced Pelvic Articulation:** The Pelvic Clock's regulated motions enable subtle pelvic articulation, which improves the pelvic region's flexibility and mobility.

9. **Basis for Pelvic Medicine:** Pelvic The Pilates clock exercise is fundamental to developing pelvic awareness, mobility, and health. It lays the groundwork for more advanced Pilates exercises.

The Pelvic Clock becomes a harmonic dance in Wall Pilates' elegant choreography, a smooth combination of pelvic mobility, core stability, attentive awareness, and supporting accuracy. The practice showcases how strength and mobility are seamlessly integrated into the Pilates journey, as the pelvis moves gently through the clock motions against the soothing wall. Pelvic Clock challenges practitioners to go on a transforming journey that shapes a harmonious body-spirit connection within the Pilates domain.

5.5: Wall Roll-Up

A fundamental exercise in Wall Pilates, the Wall Roll-Up is a skilful combination of spinal articulation and core strength. Based on Pilates' fundamentals, this exercise smoothly combines the wall's supportive embrace with the body's controlled ascent. Within the Pilates paradigm, the Wall Roll-Up becomes a transforming ritual that develops core strength, mindful movement, and a deep connection between body and breath.

1. Initial Position:

Standing with your back to the wall and your feet hip-width apart, begin the Wall Roll-Up. To provide a solid but comfortable posture, gently bend your knees. Press your hands on the wall while extending your arms upwards. With the wall as a helpful guide, this initial stance establishes a basic alignment for the following complex exercise.

2. Core Engagement and Alignment:

Ensure your spine is in a neutral posture to maintain good alignment throughout the Wall Roll-Up. To establish stability, contract your core muscles, especially your transverse abdominis. By avoiding needless effort and encouraging a smooth development of spinal articulation, alignment and core engagement provide the foundation for a controlled climb.

3. Mandated Articulatory Motions:

The dominant component of the Wall Roll-Up is the controlled articulation of the spine throughout the ascent from a standing posture to a forward fold. Start the motion with an exhale, then roll through each vertebra one at a time to enable the spine to bend and articulate forward. The wall acts as a steady support, directing the deliberate motion and improving the accuracy of the spinal articulation. As you climb, pay attention to how each vertebra engages and lifts off the wall.

4. Breathing in Time with Movement:

Breath turns become a crucial component of Wall Roll-Up. As you are ready for the exercise, take a deep breath and let your rib cage expand. Completely exhale as you start the deliberate climb using your core muscles and rolling up your spine. Breath and movement synchronization improves awareness, cultivating a mindful Pilates practice and strengthening the link between articulate spinal movement and breath.

5. Wall Assist for Managed Climb:

The wall acts as a stabilizing force for the controlled ascension during the Wall Roll-Up. The hands stay in touch with the wall, offering ongoing assistance and serving as a point of reference for proper spinal alignment. By ensuring a deliberate and progressive advancement, this support frees up practitioners to concentrate on the quality of the spinal articulation.

6. Paying Attention to Your Spine:

During the Wall Roll-Up, focus on your spine's awareness. Ascend and experience the gradual activation of each vertebra, which fosters a more complex comprehension of spinal articulation. By improving the mind-muscle connection, this conscious awareness makes it possible to feel the dynamic movement of the spine with more purpose and deliberateness.

7. Forward Fold and Complete Extension:

Aim for a complete spine extension during the Wall Roll-Up, using your core muscles to assist the upward movement. Allow your body to collapse forward at the top of the action by hinging at the hips. Do the controlled extension and forward fold to stretch and activate the whole spine fully.

8. Alignment Verification and Adjustment:

Throughout the Wall Roll-Up, check your alignment to ensure your spine stays in its sequential articulation. Adjustments may suit different people's comfort levels by changing the movement's strength or the distance from the wall. The goal is to create a transformational and uplifting ascension that is smooth and controlled.

9. Increasing Core Strength:

Throughout the exercise, the Wall Roll-Up effectively activates and strengthens the core. The core muscles play a significant role in the regulated ascent by providing strength and stability in the abdominal area. The incorporation of core strength gives the Pilates method a dynamic touch.

10. A Classy Resolution and Comeback:

The Wall Roll-Up concludes with a slow fall back to the beginning posture and a deep breath to recognize the strength and flexibility developed. Take a purposeful stance and acknowledge your newfound connection. The recovery phase is a crucial element that highlights the significance of deliberate recovery and the dynamic challenge. This thoughtful ending enhances the exercise's overall coherence and efficacy.

Wall Roll-Up Advantages:

1. **Spinal Articulation Mastery:** The Wall Roll-Up improves and masters spinal articulation, enabling each vertebra to move deliberately and sequentially.
2. **Core Strengthening**: The workout aggressively works the abdominal muscles and strengthens them, which helps to maintain general core stability.
3. **Breath-Movement Synchronization:** This technique adds to a mindful Pilates exercise by enhancing awareness and bolstering the Wall Roll-Up's fluidity.
4. **Stabilizing Wall Support:** Especially helpful for those working on spinal articulation, the wall acts as a stabilizing force, offering support for a controlled and confident execution.
5. **Mind-Body link:** A deliberate concentration on spinal awareness strengthens the link between mind and body, promoting control and elegance.
6. **Adaptable for Varied Comfort Levels**: The Wall Roll-Up is flexible enough to adjust to suit varying comfort levels and allow for increasing difficulties.

7. **Full Spinal Extension and Forward Fold:** The deliberate ascent and forward fold encourage the spine to extend, which helps to stretch and activate the whole back fully.
8. **Alignment attention:** The exercise focuses on keeping the body in the proper alignment, encouraging the best possible activation of the core muscles and reducing needless strain.
9. **Sequential Engagement of Vertebrae:** The Wall Roll-Up promotes a sophisticated awareness of spinal movement by encouraging the sequential engagement of every vertebra throughout the climb.
10. **Basis for Spinal Health:** The Wall Roll-Up is an exercise that provides the framework for future Pilates practice growth by strengthening, extending, and improving the spine's health.

The Wall Roll-Up is a dynamic ascension that appears in the elegant choreography of Wall Pilates. It is a fluid ballet of spinal articulation, core strength, conscious awareness, and supporting accuracy. The practice showcases the smooth transition between strength and flexibility in the Pilates method as the spine elegantly rises from the wall's consoling embrace. Wall Roll-Up challenges practitioners to go on a transforming journey that shapes a harmonious body-spirit connection within the Pilates domain.

5.6: Standing Side Stretch

A beautiful action in the Wall Pilates repertory, the Standing Side Stretch is a lyrical arc of core activation and spine elongation. Based on Pilates' fundamentals, this exercise smoothly combines the body's lateral stretch with the wall's supporting framework. Within the Pilates paradigm, the Standing Side Stretch becomes a transforming ritual that lengthens the spine, promotes conscious movement, and fosters a deep connection between the body and the breath.

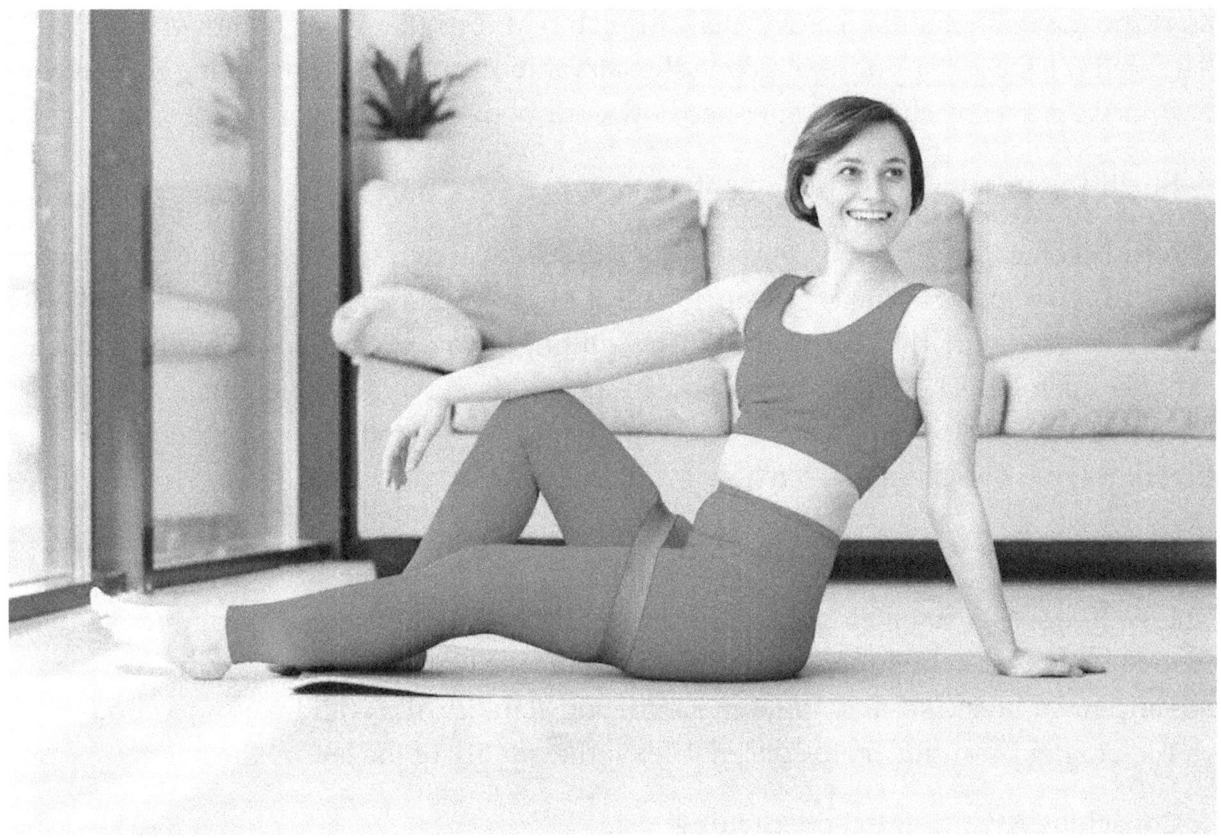

1. Initial Position:

With your side against the wall and your feet hip-width apart, begin the Standing Side Stretch. Create a stable base by bending your knees slightly to increase stability. With your fingers pointing upward, extend one arm above and push the palm against the wall. The other arm may lean slightly toward the floor or rest by your side. Starting from this posture establishes a base of alignment by using the wall as a guide to assist the next lateral stretch.

2. Core Engagement and Alignment:

When doing the Standing Side Stretch, ensure your spine is in a neutral posture to maintain good alignment. To establish stability, contract the obliques and other core muscles. By avoiding needless strain and encouraging a controlled release of tension along the side of the body, the alignment and core engagement prepare the body for the lateral stretch.

3. Motions of Lateral Flexion:

As you extend away from the wall, the lateral flexion of the spine makes the standing side stretch so effective. Leaning your upper body slightly to the side and exhaling will start the movement and create a lateral stretch that runs the whole length of your torso. The wall is a steady support, directing the lateral movement and improving the stretch's accuracy. As you reach the wall, notice how your body seems longer on the side.

4. Breathing in Time with Movement:

Breath becomes an essential component of the side stretch when standing. As you are ready for the exercise, take a deep breath and let your rib cage expand. Completely exhale as you start the lateral flexion by pulling away from the wall with your core muscles active. The coordinated breathing and movement heighten awareness, encouraging a focused Pilates practice and strengthening the breath-to-graceful-lateral-stretch link.

5. Wall Assist for Regulated Extension:

The wall acts as a stabilizing force for the regulated lateral stretch during the Standing Side Stretch. Constant support from the hand on the wall ensures a slow and deliberate advancement of the stretch. Without sacrificing stability, the wall takes on a comforting role, enabling practitioners to concentrate on the quality of the lateral flexion.

6. Conscious Attention to Lengthening:

During the Standing Side Stretch, pay close attention to how your body feels stretching. As you stretch out from the wall, notice how your whole side elongates. This cognitive awareness makes a more purposeful and intentional feeling of lateral stretch and spinal elongation possible, which strengthens the mind-muscle link.

7. Differencing Arm Positions:

Try adjusting the arm position to suit your comfort level and desired results. Try putting your arm in a new position—for example, reaching it above or letting it rest softly by your side. Every variant gives the stretch more depth and offers a chance for a unique, dynamic experience.

8. Alignment Verification and Adjustment:

Check your alignment throughout the Standing Side Stretch to ensure your spine is neutral and your lateral flexion stays controlled. Adjustments may be made to allow varying degrees of comfort by running the distance from the wall or the intensity of the stretch. The focus is on developing an empowering and freeing lateral stretch that is controlled and smooth.

9. Oblique Activation and Core Engagement:

During the lateral flexion of the Standing Side Stretch, the core muscles—especially the obliques—are actively engaged. The core must be dynamically activated to support and stabilize the spine during the controlled stretch and to encourage strength and engagement along the side of the torso.

10. A Classy Comeback and Recuperation:

The Standing Side Stretch concludes with a gradual return to an upright posture and a deep breath to recognize the extended side. Take a purposeful stance and enjoy your newfound transparency. The recovery phase is a crucial element that highlights the significance of deliberate recovery and the dynamic challenge. This thoughtful ending enhances the exercise's overall coherence and efficacy.

Aiding with Side Stretches:

1. **Lateral Flexion Mastery:** The Standing Side Stretch helps to develop and master lateral flexion, making it possible to stretch the entire side of the body purposefully and controlled.

2. **Core Engagement Enhancement:** This exercise contributes to total core strength by actively engaging and enhancing core engagement, especially by stimulating the oblique muscles.

3. **Breath-Movement Synchronization:** This technique adds to a mindful Pilates practice by enhancing awareness and sustaining the flexibility of the Standing Side Stretch.

4. **Stabilizing Wall Support:** The wall acts as a stabilizing force, supporting confident and controlled execution, especially for those practicing lateral flexion.

5. **Mind-Body Connection:** Concentrating on elongating promotes a higher

We are Creating a sensation of control and elegance throughout the activity and strengthening the mind-body connection.

1. **Adaptable for Varying Comfort Levels:** The Standing Side Stretch is flexible, allowing for adjustments to suit varying comfort levels and opportunities for increasing difficulties.

2. **Variation in Arm Positioning:** By encouraging experimentation with various arm postures, the exercise adds complexity and variety to the lateral stretch and fosters a customized experience.

3. **Alignment Emphasis:** Preserving appropriate alignment is crucial for the Standing Side Stretch as it encourages the best possible activation of the oblique muscles and reduces needless strain.

4. **Full Lengthening feeling:** The lateral flexion contributes to a thorough stretch and engagement by producing a full-lengthening feeling along the side of the body.

5. **The basis for Spinal Extension:** The Standing Side Stretch is an essential Pilates exercise that develops awareness, lengthening, and health along the side of the torso. It lays the groundwork for more advancement in the practice.

The Standing Side Stretch becomes a lyrical arc in Wall Pilates' elegant choreography, a fluid waltz of lateral flexion, core engagement, attentive awareness, and supporting accuracy. The exercise showcases the smooth transition between strength and elongation in the Pilates method as the body elegantly leans away from the wall's consoling embrace. In Pilates, Standing Side Stretch encourages practitioners to go on a transforming journey that shapes a harmonious relationship between body and soul.

5.7: Spinal Twist with Wall Support

Within the sphere of Wall Pilates, the Spinal Twist with Wall Support is an artistic exercise that promotes spinal flexibility and eases stress. Based on Pilates' fundamentals, this exercise smoothly combines the wall's supporting embrace with the spine's rotating movement. Within the Pilates paradigm, the Spinal Twist becomes a transforming ritual that promotes conscious movement, shapes spinal mobility, and deepens the connection between body and breath.

1. Initial Position:

Sitting on the floor with your side against the wall, begin the Spinal Twist. Ensure your legs are out in front of you and your spine is straight. Keeping your feet level on the ground and your knees bent, maintain a comfortable distance from the wall. Lying on your back, carefully make a 90-degree angle at your hips by swinging your legs against the wall. You may stretch your arms out to the sides so that your body forms a T. With the wall as a guide for the next rotational movement, this initial posture creates a primary alignment.

2. Core Engagement and Alignment:

Ensure your spine is in a neutral posture to maintain good alignment throughout the Spinal Twist. To establish stability, contract your core muscles, especially your transverse abdominis. Preventing undue strain and encouraging a gradual release of tension along the spine, alignment, and core engagement prepare the body for rotational action.

3. Motions in Rotation:

The core of the Spinal Twist is a deliberate twisting action produced by lowering your legs to one side and rotating your spine. Exhaling, slowly drop your knees to one side while maintaining your shoulders firmly planted on the floor to begin the action. The wall is a steady support, directing the Rotation and improving the twist's accuracy. As you rotate, notice how your spine relaxes and your back stretches gently.

4. Breathing in Time with Movement:

Breath turns become a crucial component of the spinal twist. As you are ready for the exercise, take a deep breath and let your rib cage expand. Completely release your breath as you drop your legs to one side while contracting your core muscles. Breath and movement synchronization improves consciousness, which promotes mindfulness in Pilates and strengthens the link between breath and the therapeutic spinal twist.

5. Wall Assistance for Managed Rotation:

The wall acts as a stabilizing factor to maintain the regulated rotational movement during the Spinal Twist. The legs lean lightly against the wall, giving constant support and guaranteeing a slow, deliberate twist advancement. Without sacrificing stability, the wall takes on a reassuring role, enabling practitioners to concentrate on the quality of the circular action.

6. Spinal Release with Mindful Focus:

During the Spinal Twist, direct your focused attention to the release of tension. As you bend your legs to one side, you should feel your spine relaxing and becoming more flexible and open. The mind-muscle link is improved by this cognitive awareness, enabling a more purposeful and intentional spinal twist sensation.

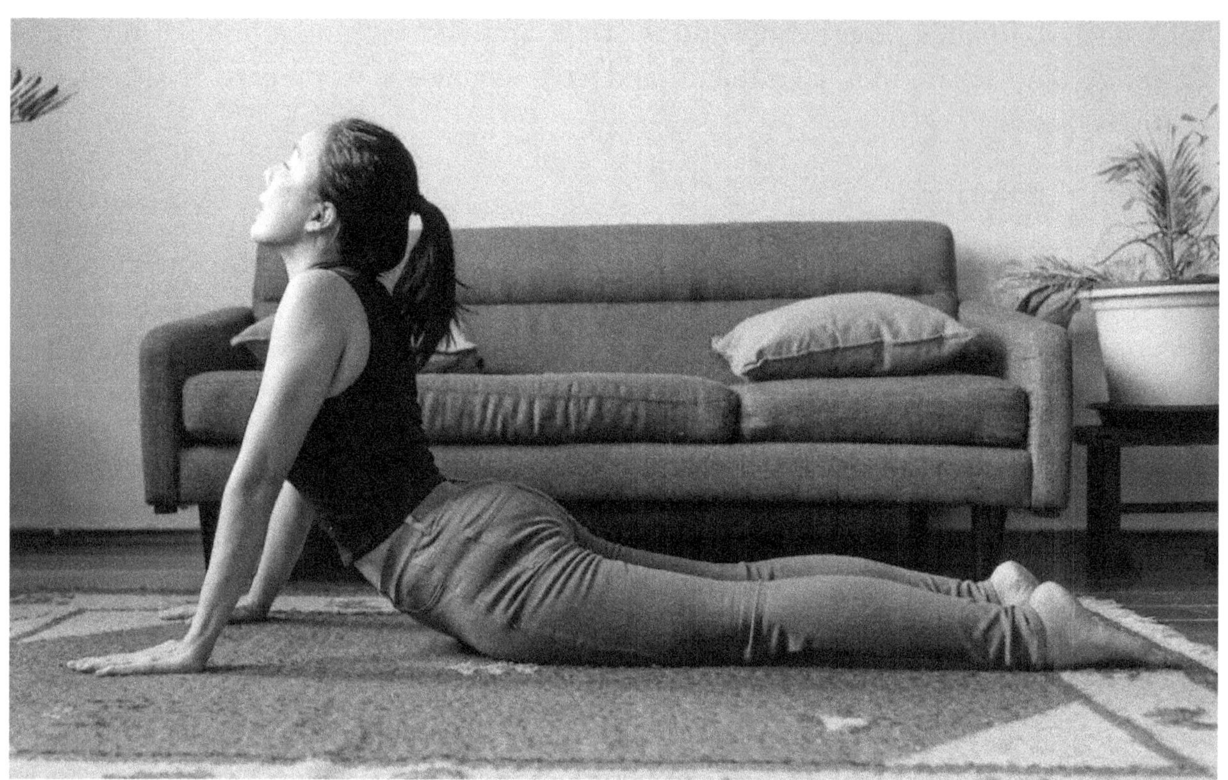

7. Difference in Leg Position:

Adjust the leg position to suit your comfort level and desired outcome while doing the twist. You may try putting your legs in various positions—for example, keeping your knees together or letting them slightly apart. Every variant deepens the twist and offers a chance for a unique, engaging experience.

8. Alignment Verification and Adjustment:

Throughout the Spinal Twist, periodically check your alignment to ensure your spine stays in its neutral Position and the rotational movement is regulated. Adjustments may suit different comfort levels by varying the twist's strength or distance from the wall. The goal is to achieve a revitalizing and uplifting spinal twist that is regulated and fluid.

9. Spinal Mobility and Core Engagement:

During the rotating action, the Spinal Twist actively engages the core muscles. The core must be dynamically activated to support and stabilize the spine during the controlled twist and enhance strength and mobility throughout the spinal column. The Pilates method gains a therapeutic component from this incorporation of core involvement.

10. A Classy Comeback and Recuperation:

Finishing the Spinal Twist is a soft return to the beginning posture and a deep breath to recognize the tension being released. Lay flat on your back and stretch your legs against the wall to realign your spine. The recovery phase is a crucial element that highlights the significance of deliberate recovery and the dynamic challenge. This thoughtful ending enhances the exercise's overall coherence and efficacy.

Spinal Twist with Wall Support Benefits:

1. **Spinal Movement Enhancement:** The Spinal Twist is a technique that improves and refines spinal movement, which permits a therapeutic and regulated stress release across the whole spine.

2. **Core Engagement and Stability:** This exercise contributes to overall core stability by actively engaging and enhancing core engagement, especially activating the transverse abdominis.

3. **Breath-Movement Synchronization:** This technique adds to a mindful Pilates practice by enhancing awareness and supporting the flexibility of the Spinal Twist.

4. **Stabilizing Wall Support:** Especially helpful for those focusing on spinal movement, the wall acts as a stabilizing force, offering support for a controlled and confident execution.

5. **Mind-Body Connection:** Concentrating on spinal release mindfully may create a more open and controlled feeling inside the practice by raising your mind-body connection.

6. **Adaptable for Varied Comfort Levels:** The Spinal Twist is flexible, allowing for adjustments to suit varying comfort levels and space for progressively more complex tasks.

7. **Variation in Leg Positioning:** This exercise promotes experimenting with various leg positions, which adds complexity and variation to the spinal twist and creates a more individualized experience.

8. **Alignment focus:** The Spinal Twist focuses on keeping the spine in the proper alignment, encouraging the best possible activation of the core muscles and reducing needless strain.

9. **Release of Tension along the Spine:** The circular movement promotes flexibility and renewal by allowing for a little release of tension along the spine.

10.   **Basis for Spinal Health:** The Spinal Twist with Wall Support is an exercise that establishes awareness, mobility, and spinal health. It also lays the groundwork for further advancements in Pilates technique.

The Spinal Twist with Wall Support, in the elegant choreography of Wall Pilates, becomes a healing experience—a fluid ballet of spinal mobility, core engagement, conscious release, and precise supporting alignment. The exercise becomes an ode to the smooth integration of strength and flexibility throughout the Pilates journey as the spine softly relaxes against the wall's welcoming embrace. Within the Pilates domain, Spinal Twist encourages practitioners to go on a transformational experience that shapes a harmonious relationship between body and soul.

Chapter 6: Flexibility and Mobility Enhancement

6.1: Wall Hamstring Stretch

One of the fundamental exercises in Wall Pilates is the Wall Hamstring Stretch, which opens the door to flexible, relaxed muscles. Based on Pilates' fundamentals, this exercise smoothly blends the wall's support with the hamstring-elongating stretch. Within the Pilates paradigm, the Wall Hamstring Stretch becomes a transformational exercise that enhances flexibility, mindful movement, and the development of a deep connection between body and breath.

1. Initial Position:

Place your back against the wall while sitting on the floor to begin the Wall Hamstring Stretch. Ensure your legs touch the wall as you extend them in front of you. Keep your back straight and use your abdominal muscles. Sit. Point your toes upwards as you flex your feet. Starting in this manner creates a base of alignment by using the wall as a guide to assist the hamstring stretch that will come next.

2. Core Engagement and Alignment:

When doing the Wall Hamstring Stretch, ensure your pelvis is firmly planted on the floor, and your spine is straight. Contract the lower abdominal muscles, in particular, to establish stability. By avoiding needless effort and encouraging a gradual release of tension throughout the hamstrings, the alignment and core engagement prepare the body for the elongating stretch.

3. Lengthening Motions:

As you extend toward your toes, the stretching motion of your hamstrings is the fundamental component of the wall hamstring stretch. Exhale to begin the action, then slowly bend at the hips to let your torso fold forward. Keep your knees slightly bent as you extend your hands toward your toes if necessary. The wall acts as a steady support, directing the stretching motion and improving the accuracy of the stretch. Examine how your hamstrings feel longer, and your legs pleasantly stretched in the back.

4. Breathing in Time with Movement:

Incorporating breath into the Wall Hamstring Stretch becomes essential. As you are ready for the exercise, take a deep breath and let your rib cage expand. Take a deep breath as you start the elongating action toward your toes using your core muscles. Breath and movement synchronization improves consciousness, which promotes mindfulness in Pilates and strengthens the link between breath and the calming hamstring stretch.

5. Wall Assistance for Regulated Extension:

The wall acts as a stabilizing force to allow for controlled extension of the hamstrings during the Wall Hamstring Stretch. The back stays in touch with the wall, giving ongoing stability and guaranteeing a slow, deliberate advancement of the stretch. Without sacrificing stability, the wall takes on a comforting role, enabling practitioners to concentrate on the quality of the elongating action.

6. Conscientious Attention to Hamstring Release:

During the Wall Hamstring Stretch, direct your focused attention to releasing tension. Stretching toward your toes will cause your hamstrings to extend, increasing your flexibility and sensation of openness. By improving the mind-muscle connection, this cognitive awareness makes it possible to feel the hamstring stretch more purposefully and deliberately.

7. Differencing Hand Positions:

Try adjusting the hand placement to suit your comfort level and desired results. You may put your hands in other places, such as your shins, ankles, or even your yoga strap, for more support. Every variant gives the stretch more depth and offers a chance for a unique, dynamic experience.

8. Alignment Verification and Adjustment:

Check your alignment periodically while doing the Wall Hamstring Stretch to ensure your spine stays straight and the elongating action is controlled. Adjustments may be made to allow varying degrees of comfort by running the distance from the wall or the intensity of the stretch. The focus is on developing an empowering and freeing stretch for the hamstrings that is controlled and flowing.

9. Flexibility of the Lower Body and Core Engagement:

The Wall Hamstring Stretch aggressively works the core muscles, especially the lower abdominals, throughout the elongating action. For the controlled stretch to be effective, the lower back and hamstrings must be strengthened and stabilized, which calls for dynamic core activation. The Pilates method gains a therapeutic component from this incorporation of core involvement.

10. A Classy Comeback and Recuperation:

The Wall Hamstring Stretch ends with a soft return to the beginning posture and a deep breath to recognize the release of tension. With purpose, sit up straight, enjoying your newfound freedom. The recovery phase is a crucial element that highlights the significance of deliberate recovery and the dynamic challenge. This thoughtful ending enhances the exercise's overall coherence and efficacy.

Advantages of Wall Hamstring Extension:

1. **Enhancement of Hamstring Flexibility:** The Wall Hamstring Stretch works to fine-tune and amplify the flexibility of the hamstrings, which permits a therapeutic and controlled release of tension down the back of the legs.

2. **Core Engagement and Stability:** This exercise contributes to overall core stability by actively engaging and enhancing core engagement, especially activating the lower abdominals.

3. **Breath-Movement Synchronization:** This technique adds to a mindful Pilates practice by promoting awareness and the flexibility of the Hamstring Stretch.

4. **Stabilizing Wall Support:** The wall acts as a stabilizing force, supporting those working on hamstring flexibility and offering support for a controlled and confident execution.

5. **Mind-Body Connection:** Concentrating on hamstring release with awareness increases the mind-body connection and creates an open and controlled feeling throughout the practice.

6. **Adaptable for Varying Comfort Levels:** The Wall Hamstring Stretch is flexible, allowing for adjustments to suit varying comfort levels and opportunities for increasing difficulties.

7. **Variation in Hand Positioning:** By encouraging experimentation with various hand positions, the exercise adds complexity and variation to the hamstring stretch and fosters a customized experience.

8. **Alignment Emphasis:** The Wall Hamstring Stretch strongly emphasizes maintaining appropriate alignment to maximize core muscle activation and minimize needless strain.

9. **Release of Tension along the Hamstrings:** The elongating action promotes flexibility and a sensation of renewal by allowing for a mild release of tension along the hamstrings.

10. **Basis for Flexibility in the Lower Body:** The Wall Hamstring Stretch is a fundamental exercise that prepares the body for future advancement in Pilates practice by increasing awareness, flexibility, and health in the lower back and hamstrings.

The Wall Hamstring Stretch is a doorway that leads to a smooth journey of hamstring flexibility, core engagement, mindful release, and supporting accuracy in the elegant dance of Wall Pilates. The exercise shows how well flexibility and strength are integrated into the Pilates method as the body extends elegantly toward the wall. In Pilates, Wall Hamstring Stretch encourages practitioners to go on a transforming journey that shapes a harmonious connection between body and soul.

6.2: Side Leg Lift and Hold

The Side Leg Lift and Hold is a sophisticated exercise that sculpts hip strength and stability with elegance and precision. It is a jewel in the Wall Pilates repertory. Based on Pilates' fundamentals, this exercise skillfully blends the difficulty of raising and holding the leg in a lateral posture with the wall's support. Within the Pilates paradigm, the Side Leg Lift and Hold develops into a transformational exercise that strengthens the hips, encourages conscious movement, and deepens the connection between the body and the breath.

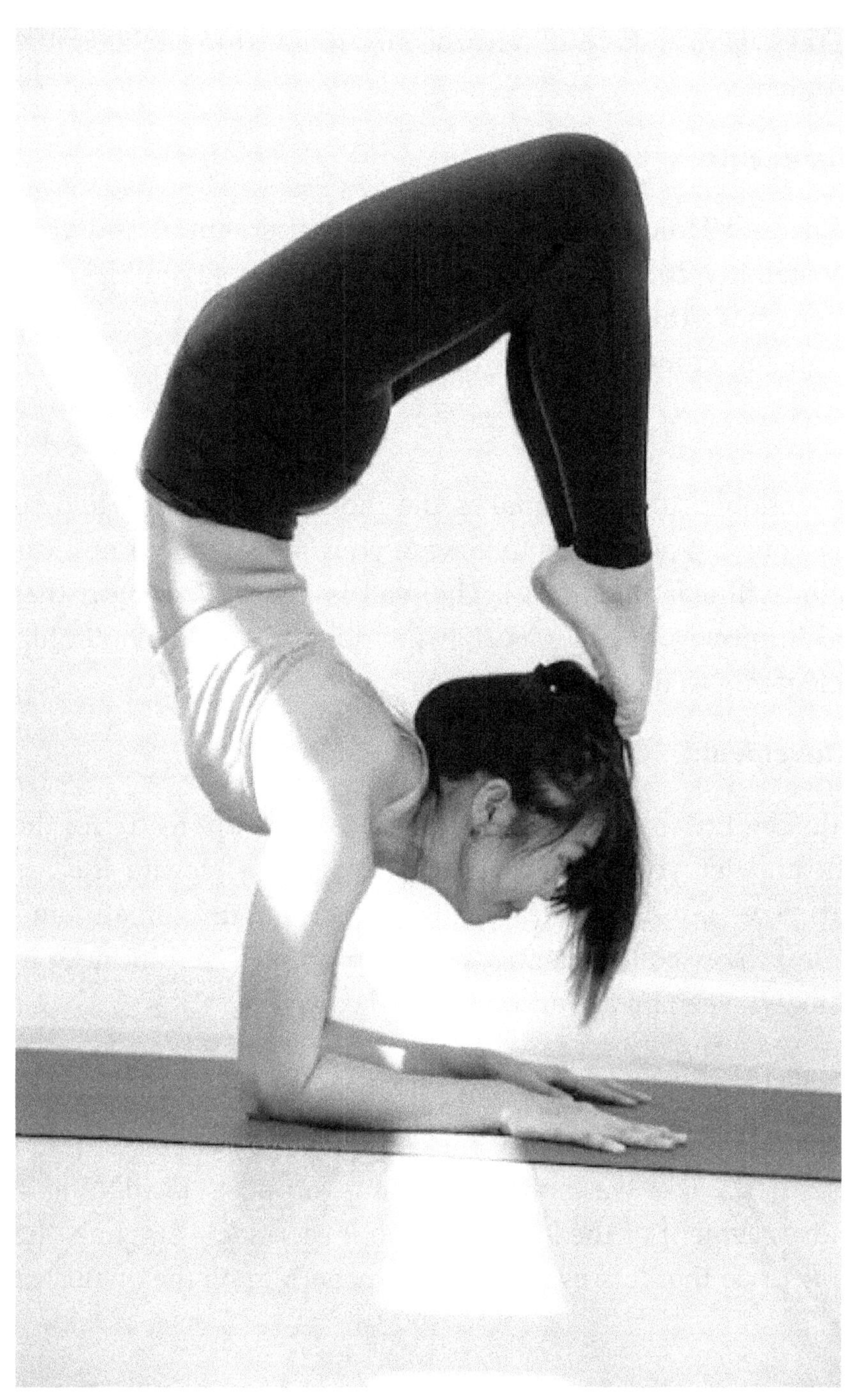

1. Initial Position:

Standing on your side facing the wall, begin the Side Leg Lift and Hold. Maintain a straight, tall posture and space your feet hip-width apart to ensure correct alignment. For balance, place one hand gently on the wall while bending the supporting leg slightly. With toes pointing, the opposite leg—the one that has to be lifted—should be straight and stretched. With the wall as a helpful reference for the next task, this initial stance creates a primary alignment.

2. Core Engagement and Alignment:

When doing the Side Leg Lift and Hold, make sure your pelvis is neutral and your spine is straight. To establish stability, contract the obliques and other core muscles. The alignment and core engagement make the lateral leg lift possible, promoting a regulated activation of the hip muscles and avoiding needless strain.

3. Elevating Motion:

The leg's deliberate raising motion to the side makes the Side Leg Lift and Hold so effective. Exhaling and using your hip abductors to elevate your leg laterally until it is at or slightly above hip height will start the action. The wall is a steady support that directs the lifting motion and improves lift accuracy. Pay attention to how the outer hip muscles feel as the leg rises elegantly to the side.

4. Breathing in Time with Movement:

A vital component of the Side Leg Lift and Hold is breathing. As you are ready for the exercise, take a deep breath and let your rib cage expand. As you elevate the leg laterally and contract your core muscles, release the whole breath. Breath and movement synchronization improves consciousness, which promotes mindfulness in Pilates and strengthens the link between breath and the complex leg lift.

5. Supporting the Wall for Stability:

The wall stabilizes the body's balance and stability throughout the Side Leg Lift and Hold. The hand softly resting on the wall offers ongoing support, facilitating a deliberate and progressive advancement of the leg lift. Without sacrificing stability, the wall takes on a comforting presence that lets practitioners concentrate on the quality of the lifting motion.

6. Phase of Holding:

Hold the leg firm for the predetermined amount of time when it has reached its elevated position. This holding phase is an essential component that ups the difficulty and calls for continuous hip muscular activation. By helping to maintain stability, the wall support frees practitioners to concentrate on the isometric contraction and attentive management of the maintained posture.

7. Concise Attention to Hip Activation:

Pay close attention to how the hip muscles contract throughout the lifting and holding stages. To hold the leg up and manage the action, feel the outer hip muscles cooperating. By improving the mind-muscle connection, this conscious awareness makes it possible to feel hip strength more purposefully and intentionally.

8. Difference in Leg Position:

Try adjusting the leg position to suit your comfort level and objectives. Try other leg locations, such as varying the lift height or adding little pulses during the holding period. Every variant gives the workout more depth and offers a chance for a unique, dynamic experience.

9. Alignment Verification and Adjustment:

Check your alignment periodically while doing the Side Leg Lift and Hold to ensure your spine stays straight and the lifting motion is controlled. Adjustments may suit varying degrees of comfort by changing the lift's intensity or distance from the wall. The goal is to create a leg lift that is controlled and fluid, which will contour the hips and feel empowered.

10. Calm Lowering and Recuperation:

The Side Leg Lift and Hold concludes with a graceful lowering of the raised leg and a deep breath to signify the challenge's accomplishment. With purpose, stand up straight and acknowledge the power and engagement in your hips. The recovery phase is a crucial element that highlights the significance of deliberate recovery and the dynamic challenge. This thoughtful ending enhances the exercise's overall coherence and efficacy.

Advantages of the Side Leg Lift and Hold:

1. **Improving Hip Strength:** This exercise, focusing mainly on the abductors, improves hip strength and overall hip stability.
2. **Core Engagement and Stability:** This exercise aggressively works the core, particularly the obliques, which helps to maintain stability throughout the leg lift.
3. **Breath-Movement Synchronization:** This technique adds to a mindful Pilates exercise by enhancing awareness and sustaining the fluidity of the Side Leg Lift and Hold.
4. **Stabilizing Wall Support:** The wall is a stabilizing force for those focusing on hip strength, offering support for a controlled and confident execution.

5. **Mind-Body Connection:** Attention to hip activation with awareness increases the mind-body connection and develops a stronger, more controlled feeling throughout the activity.

6. **Adaptable for Varied Comfort Levels:** The Side Leg Lift and Hold are flexible, allowing adjustments to suit varying degrees of comfort and space for progressively more complex tasks.

7. **Variation in Leg Positioning:** The exercise adds complexity and variety to the hip challenge and fosters a customized experience by encouraging experimentation with various leg postures.

8. **Alignment Emphasis:** The Side Leg Lift and Hold strongly emphasize maintaining appropriate alignment to maximize hip muscle activation and minimize needless strain.

9. **Isometric Challenge in Holding Phase:** This isometric challenge, which requires continuous hip muscular activation, is introduced during the holding phase and helps build muscle endurance.

10. **The Basis for Hip Sculpture:** The Side Leg Lift and Hold is an essential Pilates exercise that develops hip awareness, strength, and definition. It also lays the groundwork for more advanced Pilates techniques.

The Side Leg Lift and Hold is a beautiful action that demonstrates hip strength, stability, conscious engagement, and supporting accuracy in the elegant choreography of Wall Pilates. The exercise demonstrates the smooth fusion of power and grace in the Pilates journey as the leg raises gently against the wall's soothing embrace. Within the Pilates domain, Side Leg Lift and Hold enables practitioners to go on a transformational excursion that shapes a harmonious relationship between body and soul.

6.3: Wall Pigeon Pose

A fascinating addition to the repertoire of Wall Pilates, the Wall Pigeon Pose develops hip flexibility and promotes a thoughtful release. Based on Pilates' fundamentals, this exercise skillfully blends the wall's support with the stretching and opening of the hip muscles. Within the Pilates paradigm, the Wall Pigeon Pose becomes a transformational journey that enhances hip flexibility, mindful movement, and the development of a deep connection between body and breath.

1. Initial Position:

From a reasonable distance away, face the wall to begin the Wall Pigeon Pose. With your arms extended shoulder-high, place your hands on the wall for support. Firmly plant one foot on the ground, bend the other knee, and raise the foot toward the wall. This creates a shape similar to the yoga Pigeon Pose, as the raised knee and shin are encouraged to rest comfortably on the wall. With the wall acting as a guide for support, this beginning posture creates a basic alignment for the next hip-opening stretch.

2. Core Engagement and Alignment:

Ensure your hips are squared to the wall to maintain good posture in the Wall Pigeon Pose. To keep the spine and stabilize the pelvis, contract your core muscles. The hip-opening stretch is made possible by the alignment and core engagement, which also help to minimize undue strain and encourage a gradual release of tension along the hip muscles.

3. Opening the Hips Stretch:

The gradual opening and stretching of the hip muscles is the foundation of the Wall Pigeon Pose. The elevated leg feels more prolonged and more relaxed as the hip of the extended leg expands outward and the shin and knee press against the wall. The wall is steady support, directing the stretching motion and improving the hip release's accuracy. Examine how the hip muscles feel as they progressively give way to the stretch and as you consciously let go of any stored tension.

4. Breathing in Time with Movement:

Breath becomes a necessary component of Wall Pigeon Pose. As you prepare for the stretch, take a deep breath and let your rib cage expand. Fully exhale as you let go of the hip-opening action and contract your core muscles. Breath and movement in unison improve awareness, cultivating a mindful Pilates practice and strengthening the link between breath and the therapeutic hip stretch.

5. Mildly Compressive Wall Support:

The wall offers a little compression on the raised hip during Wall Pigeon Pose, intensifying the stretch and producing a reassuring sense. By encouraging a slow and deliberate increase in the stretch, this support enables practitioners to explore the hip release's depth without jeopardizing their stability.

6. Concise Attention to Hip Release:

During Wall Pigeon Pose, direct your conscious attention to releasing tension. You may feel your hips opening up and your muscles extending as you give yourself up to the wall's support. By improving the mind-muscle connection, this conscious awareness makes it possible to feel hip flexibility and release more purposefully and intentionally.

7. Knee Height Variation:

Adjust the height of the elevated knee to suit your comfort level and desired results. The knee may be positioned higher or lower depending on how far the foot is from the wall. Every variant gives the stretch more depth and offers a chance for a unique, dynamic experience.

8. Alignment Verification and Adjustment:

In Wall Pigeon Pose, periodically verify that your hips stay square to the wall and that the stretching action is controlled. Adjustments may be made to different comfort levels, adjusting the height of the elevated knee or the distance from the wall. The goal is to achieve a freeing and revitalizing, controlled, and flowing hip-opening stretch.

9. Mindful Surrender and Core Engagement:

To stabilize the spine and pelvis in the Wall Pigeon Pose, contract your core muscles. By engaging the core consciously, one may succumb to the hip-opening stretch with awareness, striking a balance between strength and relaxation. The Pilates method gains a therapeutic component from this incorporation of core involvement.

10. Smooth Shift and Recuperation:

Finishing the Wall In Pigeon Pose, one should gently move away from the wall and take a deep breath to recognize the release of tension. Take a deliberate step back and enjoy your newly acquired hip suppleness. The recovery phase is a crucial element that highlights the significance of intentional recovery and the dynamic challenge. This thoughtful ending enhances the exercise's overall coherence and efficacy.

Wall Pigeon Pose Benefits:

1. **Enhancing Hip Flexibility**: The Wall Pigeon Pose honed and improved hip flexibility, enabling a therapeutic and regulated release of tension along the hip muscles.

2. **Core Engagement and Stability:** During the hip-opening stretch, the exercise actively engages and strengthens core engagement, which helps to provide general stability and support.

3. **Breath-Movement Synchronization:** This technique adds to a mindful Pilates exercise by promoting awareness and maintaining the flexibility of the Pigeon Pose.

4. **Soft Compression for Support:** The wall softly compresses the elevated hip, improving the stretch and producing a reassuring feeling when the hip is released.

5. **Mind-Body Connection:** Paying attention to the release of the hips with mindfulness increases the mind-body connection and creates an open and controlled feeling throughout the exercise.

6. **Adaptable for Varied Comfort Levels:** The Wall Pigeon Pose is flexible, allowing for adjustments to suit varying degrees of comfort and opportunities for increasing difficulties.

7. **Difference in Knee Height:** This exercise promotes experimenting with various knee heights, which adds complexity and variety to the hip stretch and fosters a customized experience.

8. **Alignment Emphasis:** The Wall Pigeon Pose emphasizes alignment to reduce needless strain and promote optimum core muscle activation.

9. **Gentle Stretch for Hip Release:** This stretching technique helps to promote flexibility and a feeling of renewal by gently releasing tension along the hip muscles.

10. **Basis for Hip Health:** Wall Pigeon Pose is an essential exercise that develops hip awareness, flexibility, and health. It also lays the groundwork for further Pilates practice growth.

The Wall Pigeon Pose becomes a gentle journey of hip flexibility, conscious release, and supporting accuracy in Wall Pilates' elegant choreography. The exercise is testimony to the seamless integration of flexibility and conscious connection within the Pilates journey as the hip releases elegantly against the wall's welcoming embrace. In Pilates, Wall Pigeon Pose enables practitioners to transform, creating a harmonious connection between body and soul.

6.4: Standing Figure Four Stretch

In the world of Wall Pilates, the Standing Figure Four Stretch is a compelling position that delicately uses the wall's supporting force to balance strength and flexibility. Based on Pilates' fundamentals, this exercise combines the hip muscles' dynamic stretch with the wall's support for stability. Within the Pilates paradigm, the Standing Figure Four Stretch develops as a transformational practice that enhances hip flexibility, mindful movement, and the development of a deep connection between body and breath.

1. Initial Position:

Start the Standing Figure Four Stretch by positioning yourself comfortably away from the wall and facing it. Place both hands at shoulder height on the wall to maintain a tall and straight posture. While keeping your other foot elevated off the ground, shift your weight onto one leg. Forming a figure-four with the ankle just above the knee, cross the elevated leg across the standing leg. With the wall acting as a guide for support, this beginning posture creates a basic alignment for the next hip-opening stretch.

2. Core Engagement and Alignment:

Make sure your hips are squared to the wall to maintain good alignment while doing the Standing Figure Four Stretch. To keep the spine and stabilize the pelvis, contract your core muscles. The dynamic stretch is made possible by the alignment and core engagement, promoting a regulated release of tension along the hip muscles and avoiding needless strain.

3. Opening the Hips Stretch:

The Standing Figure Four's main points The act of intentionally opening and extending the hip muscles is known as stretch. The elevated leg's hip expands outward while the crossed leg rests on the opposing thigh, boosting and relieving tension. The wall is steady support, directing the stretching motion and improving the hip release's accuracy. Examine how the hip muscles feel as they progressively give way to the stretch and as you consciously let go of any stored tension.

4. Breathing in Time with Movement:

Breath becomes an essential component of the Figure Four Standing Stretch. As you prepare for the stretch, take a deep breath and let your rib cage expand. Fully exhale as you let go of the hip-opening action and contract your core muscles. Breath and movement in unison improve awareness, cultivating a mindful Pilates practice and strengthening the link between breath and the therapeutic hip stretch.

5. Wall assistance for Balance:

The wall offers crucial assistance for maintaining Balance during the Standing Figure Four Stretch. The stability provided by the hands resting on the wall enables a slow and deliberate advancement of the stretch. Without sacrificing strength, the wall takes on a comforting role, allowing practitioners to concentrate on the quality of the stretching exercise.

6. Concise Attention to Hip Release:

Concentrate intently on letting go of tension while doing the Standing Figure 4 stretch. You may feel your hips opening up and your muscles extending as you give yourself up to the wall's support. By improving the mind-muscle connection, this conscious awareness makes it possible to feel hip flexibility and release more purposefully and intentionally.

7. The difference in Leg Position:

Examine different crossed-leg heights to customize the stretch to your comfort level and desired results. One may modify the figure-four posture by adjusting the foot's positioning on the standing leg. Every variant gives the stretch more depth and offers a chance for a unique, dynamic experience.

8. Alignment Verification and Adjustment:

Throughout the Standing Figure Four Stretch, ensure your hips stay square to the wall and that the stretching motion is controlled by periodically checking your alignment. Adjustments may be made to suit different comfort levels by varying the height of the crossed leg or the distance from the wall. The goal is to achieve a freeing and revitalizing, controlled, and flowing hip-opening stretch.

9. Mindful Surrender and Core Engagement:

To stabilize the spine and pelvis during the Standing Figure Four Stretch, contract your core muscles. By engaging the core consciously, one may succumb to the hip-opening stretch with awareness, striking a balance between strength and relaxation. The Pilates method gains a therapeutic component from this incorporation of core involvement.

10. Smooth Shift and Recuperation:

The Standing Figure Four's Conclusion Stretching entails releasing the crossed leg gracefully and taking a deep breath to recognize the tension being released. Take a deliberate step back and enjoy your newly acquired hip suppleness. The recovery phase is a crucial element that highlights the significance of intentional recovery and the dynamic challenge. This thoughtful ending enhances the exercise's overall coherence and efficacy.

Advantages of Figure Four Stretch Standing:

1. **Hip Flexibility Enhancement**: The Standing Figure Four Stretch facilitates a therapeutic and regulated release of tension along the hip muscles by perfecting and amplifying hip flexibility.

2. **Core Engagement and Stability:** During the hip-opening stretch, the exercise actively engages and strengthens core engagement, which helps to provide general stability and support.

3. **Breath-Movement Synchronization:** This technique adds to a mindful Pilates practice by enhancing awareness and sustaining the fluidity of the Figure Four Stretch.

4. **Wall Support for Balance:** By providing crucial support for preserving Balance during the stretch, the wall frees practitioners to concentrate on the caliber of their stretching technique.

5. **Mind-Body Connection:** Paying attention to the release of the hips with mindfulness increases the mind-body connection and creates an open and controlled feeling throughout the exercise.

6. **Adaptable for Varied Comfort Levels:** The Standing Figure Four Stretch is flexible, accommodating adjustments to suit varying degrees of comfort and opportunities for increasing difficulty levels.

7. **Variation in Leg Positioning:** This exercise promotes experimenting with various leg positions, which adds complexity and variety to the hip stretch and creates a more individualized experience.

8. **Alignment Emphasis:** The Standing Figure Four Stretch emphasizes keeping the body in the proper alignment, encouraging the best possible activation of the core muscles and reducing needless strain.

9. **Therapeutic Release of Hip Tension:** Stretching helps relieve hip muscle tension, promoting flexibility and a feeling of renewal.

10. **Equilibrated Power and Flexibility:** Figure Four Standing Stretch is a valuable addition to the Pilates repertory because it strikes a harmonic balance between strength and flexibility.

The Standing Figure Four Stretch becomes a dance in Wall Pilates' elegant choreography, a fluid fusion of strength, flexibility, conscious connection, and precise support. The exercise becomes a monument to the harmonious flow of the Pilates journey as the hip yields effortlessly to the wall's warm embrace. In Pilates, Standing Figure Four Stretch encourages practitioners to go on a transforming journey that shapes a harmonious relationship between body and soul.

6.5: Wall-Assisted Split Stretch

A fascinating posture in Wall Pilates, the Wall-Assisted Split Stretch is a dynamic exercise that releases lower body flexibility while maintaining grace and elegance. Based on the basic principles of Pilates, this stretch combines the difficulty of achieving a split posture with the wall's support. Within the Pilates paradigm, the Wall-Assisted Split Stretch becomes a transformational exercise that builds a strong connection between body and breath, promotes mindful movement, and stretches the hips and hamstrings.

1. Initial Position:

Faced toward the wall and standing at a modest distance, begin the Wall-Assisted Split Stretch. Place both hands at shoulder height on the wall to maintain a tall and straight posture. Raise a leg and put it straight out in front of you. The split posture is started by extending the opposite leg backwards. The split begins with an emphasis on maintaining alignment and balance, with the hands on the wall providing initial support. This first Position creates a base of alignment by using the wall as a guide to support the next stretch.

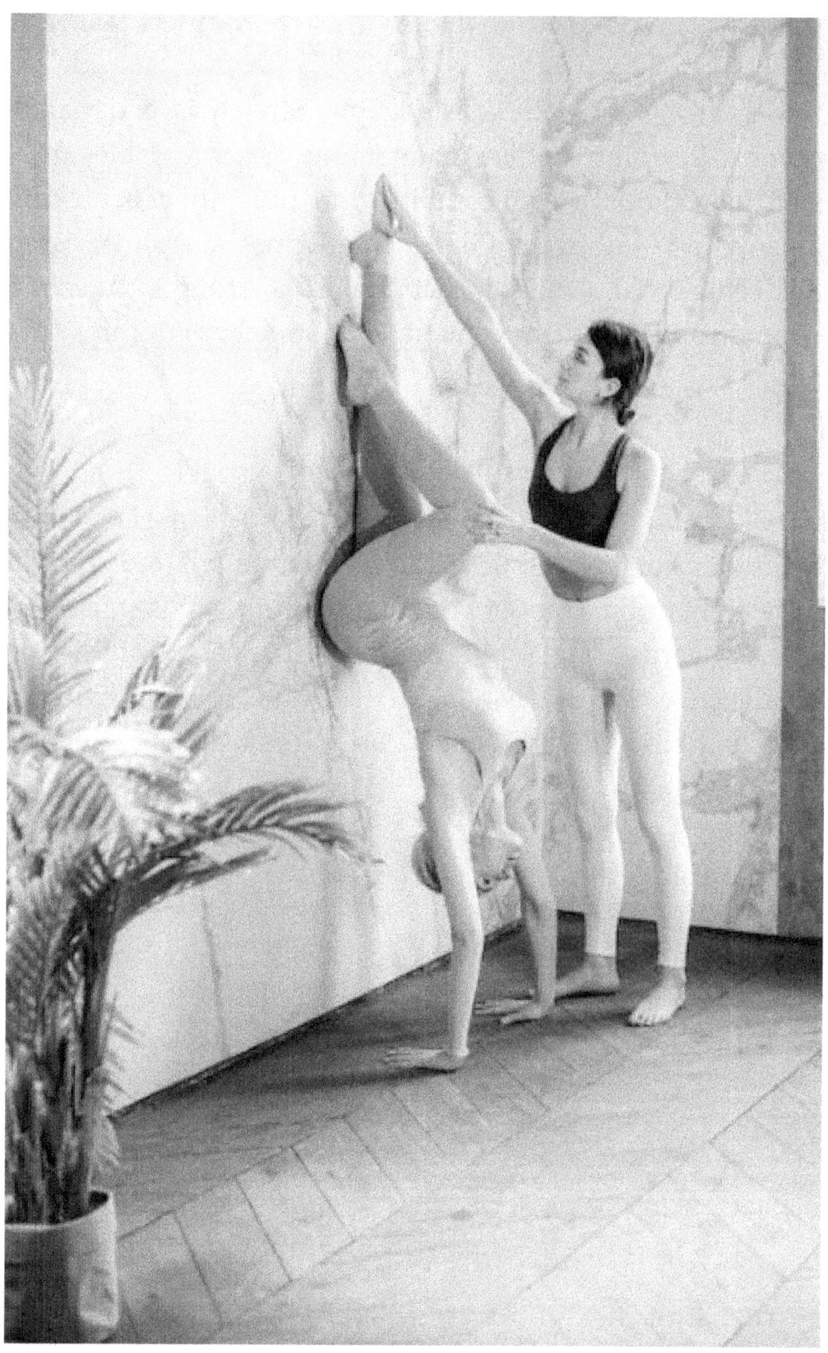

2. Core Engagement and Alignment:

Ensure your hips are squared to the wall to maintain good alignment throughout the Wall-Assisted Split Stretch. To keep the spine and stabilize the pelvis, contract your core muscles. The dynamic split stretch is made possible by the alignment and core engagement, which also help to promote regulated movement through the lower body and avoid needless strain.

3. Motion of a Dynamic Split:

Achieving and deepening the split stance via dynamic movement is the core of the Wall-Assisted Split Stretch. The wall offers crucial stability and balancing support as the split deepens. To create a feeling of stretch and openness, the split includes purposefully stretching the hamstrings and hip flexors. Because it acts as a continuous guidance, the wall helps practitioners explore the depth of their flexibility with control and improves the accuracy of the split movement.

4. Breathing in Time with Movement:

Breath becomes an essential component of the Split Stretch with Wall Assistance. As you prepare for the stretch, take a deep breath and let your rib cage expand. Completely exhale as you relax into the split posture using your core muscles. Breath and movement synchronization improves awareness, cultivating a mindful Pilates practice and strengthening the breath-to-dynamic lower body stretch relationship.

5. Balance and Alignment Wall Support:

The wall is essential in the Wall-Assisted Split Stretch because it supports the body while preserving alignment and balance. A slow and controlled advancement in the split is possible because of the stability of the hands resting on the wall. Without sacrificing strength, the wall takes on a comforting role, allowing practitioners to concentrate on the quality of the stretching exercise.

6. Pay Attention to Your Lower Body's Flexibility:

During the Wall-Assisted Split Stretch, pay close attention to how flexible your lower body is. As you investigate the depth of the split, notice how your hip flexors and hamstrings gradually extend. By improving the mind-muscle link, this cognitive awareness makes it possible to feel lower body flexibility more purposefully and intentionally.

7. Difference in Divided Depth:

Try varying the split's depth to make the stretch more comfortable and beneficial for your objectives. It is possible to change the split Position by adjusting the foot's distance from the wall. Every variant gives the stretch more depth and offers a chance for a unique, dynamic experience.

8. Alignment Verification and Adjustment:

Ensure your hips stay square to the wall, and the split movement is controlled by periodically checking your alignment throughout the Wall-Assisted Split Stretch. Adjustments may suit different people's comfort levels by varying the split's depth or distance from the wall. The focus is on achieving a liberated and powerful lower body stretch that is controlled and flowing.

9. Mindful Stretching and Core Engagement: To support the spine and pelvis, engage your core muscles throughout the Wall-Assisted Split Stretch. By consciously engaging the core, one may mindfully extend the lower body, striking a balance between strength and relaxation. Incorporating core engagement gives the Pilates exercise a dynamic quality and encourages comprehensive flexibility development.

10. Smooth Shift and Recuperation:

The Wall-Assisted Split Stretch concludes with a smooth release from the split posture and a deep breath to recognize the stretch's profundity. With purpose, stand up straight and enjoy your newly acquired lower body flexibility. The recovery phase is a crucial element that highlights the significance of deliberate recovery and the dynamic challenge. This thoughtful ending enhances the exercise's overall coherence and efficacy.

Wall-Assisted Split Stretch Benefits:

1. **Improving Lower Body Flexibility**: The Wall-Assisted Split Stretch improves lower body flexibility, facilitating a dynamic and controlled release of tension in the hamstrings and hip flexors.

2. **Core Engagement and Stability:** During the dynamic split stretch, the exercise aggressively engages and strengthens core engagement, which helps to provide general stability and support.

3. **Breath-Movement Synchronization:** This technique adds to a mindful Pilates exercise by enhancing awareness and sustaining the fluidity of the Wall-Assisted Split Stretch. To maintain balance and alignment throughout the split, practitioners may concentrate on the quality of the stretching action thanks to the wall's vital support.

4. **Mind-Body Connection:** Paying attention to lower body flexibility with mindfulness increases the mind-body connection and creates an open and controlled feeling throughout the workout.

5. **Adaptable for Varied Flexibility Levels:** The Wall-Assisted Split Stretch is flexible, allowing for adjustments to suit varying degrees of flexibility and opportunities for increasing difficulties.

6. **Difference in Split Depth:** This exercise promotes experimenting with various split depths, which adds complexity and variety to the lower body stretch and fosters a customized experience.

7. **Alignment Emphasis:** The Wall-Assisted Split Stretch emphasizes keeping the body in alignment, encouraging the best possible engagement of the core muscles and avoiding needless strain.

8. **Dynamic Lower Body Stretch:** This stretching exercise releases tension dynamically along the hamstrings and hip flexors, which helps to create a feeling of empowerment and release.

9. **Integration of Strength and Flexibility:** The Wall-Assisted Split Stretch is a valuable addition to the Pilates repertory since it successfully integrates strength and flexibility.

The Wall-Assisted Split Stretch becomes a dance in Wall Pilates' elegant choreography, a fluid fusion of strength, flexibility, conscious connection, and precise support. This exercise demonstrates the smooth harmony of the Pilates method as the lower body unfurls smoothly against the wall's soothing embrace. Wall-Assisted Split Stretch is a Pilates exercise that encourages practitioners to explore transformation and create a harmonious connection between body and soul.

6.6: Quadriceps Stretch Using Wall

Within Wall Pilates, the Quadriceps Stretch Using Wall is a revitalizing exercise that uses the wall's support to liberate flexibility in the front legs. Based on the core principles of Pilates, this stretch smoothly combines the dynamic release of tension in the quadriceps with the stabilizing effect of the wall. Within the Pilates paradigm, the Quadriceps Stretch Using the Wall transforms the front leg muscles, encourages mindful movement, and develops a deep connection between body and breath.

1. Initial Position:

Starting with your side against the wall, make sure you are at a comfortable distance to begin the quadriceps stretch. Keeping your posture tall and straight, place one hand at shoulder height on the wall for support. Lift the heel toward the glutes by bending the knee of the leg closest to the wall. To gently bend the knee, grasp the ankle with the hand on the same side. With the wall acting as a reference for support, this beginning posture creates a basic alignment for the next quadriceps stretch.

2. Core Engagement and Alignment:

When doing the quadriceps stretch, ensure your leg is straight and your knee is just behind your hip to maintain correct alignment. To keep the spine and stabilize the pelvis, contract your core muscles. The alignment and core engagement make the dynamic stretch possible, which promotes regulated movement through the quadriceps and avoids needless strain.

3. Active Quadriceps Extension:

Pulling the heel softly towards the glutes is a dynamic exercise that is the core of the Quadriceps. Stretch Using the Wall. The wall offers crucial stability and balancing support, enabling a slow and steady increase in the stretch. The purpose of the stretch is to intentionally release tension in the quadriceps, which results in a feeling of flexibility and elongation. Because it acts as a steady guide, the wall helps practitioners explore the depth of their flexibility with control and improves the accuracy of the stretching action.

4. Breathing in Time with Movement:

A vital component of the quadriceps stretch is breathing. As you prepare for the stretch, take a deep breath and let your rib cage expand. Pull the heel toward the glutes and completely exhale as you contract your core muscles. Breath and movement in unison improve awareness, cultivating a mindful Pilates practice and strengthening the link between breath and the therapeutic quadriceps stretch.

5. Wall Support for Stability: The wall is an essential source of support for balance and stability during the Quadriceps Stretch Using Wall exercise. The hand resting on the wall provides a point of touch, enabling a slow and deliberate movement throughout the stretch. Without sacrificing stability, the wall takes on a comforting role, allowing practitioners to concentrate on the quality of the stretching exercise.

6. A Concise Concentration on Quadriceps Release:

During the stretch, pay close attention to the quadriceps' release of tension. Pull the heel slowly toward the glutes, feeling the muscle gradually lengthen. By improving the mind-muscle connection, this cognitive awareness makes it possible to feel quadriceps flexibility more purposefully and intentionally.

7. Difference in Intensity of Stretch:

Try varying the stretch's intensity to make it more comfortable and meet your objectives. To run the amount of stretch, you may change the heel's height and how far away it is from the wall. Every variant gives the stretch more depth and offers a chance for a unique, dynamic experience.

8. Alignment Verification and Adjustment:

Ensure your standing leg stays straight and the stretch action is controlled by periodically checking your alignment while doing the quadriceps stretch. Adjustments may be made to suit different comfort levels by varying the heel height or the distance from the wall. The goal is to achieve a freeing and revitalizing quadriceps stretch that is controlled and flowing.

9. Conscious Stretching and Core Engagement:

To stabilize the spine and pelvis during the quadriceps stretch, contract your core muscles. By engaging the core consciously, one may try the quadriceps mindfully, striking a balance between strength and release. By including core involvement, Pilates becomes more therapeutic and encourages a comprehensive approach to flexibility.

10. Smooth Shift and Recuperation:

The last step in the quadriceps stretch is to release the heel gracefully and take a deep breath to recognize the release of tension. With purpose, stand up straight and enjoy the flexibility of your newly developed quadriceps. The recovery phase is a crucial element that highlights the significance of deliberate recovery and the dynamic challenge. This thoughtful ending enhances the exercise's overall coherence and efficacy.

Advantages of Wall-Based Quadriceps Stretching

1. **Enhanced Quadriceps Flexibility**: This exercise honed and improved quadriceps flexibility, enabling a dynamic and controlled stress release.

2. **Core Engagement and Stability:** During the dynamic stretch, the quadriceps stretch actively engages and strengthens core engagement, which helps to provide general stability and support.

3. **Breath-Movement Synchronization:** This technique adds to a mindful Pilates exercise by enhancing awareness and sustaining the stretch's smoothness.

4. **Wall Support for Stability:** The wall gives practitioners the necessary support to maintain their balance and stability during the stretch, enabling them to concentrate on the form of the stretch.

5. **Mind-Body Connection:** Paying attention to the release of the quadriceps with mindfulness increases the mind-body connection and creates an open and controlled feeling throughout the exercise.

6. **Adaptable for Varied Flexibility Levels**: The Quadriceps Stretch Using Wall is flexible, allowing for adjustments to suit varying degrees of flexibility and opportunities for increasing difficulties.

7. **The difference in Stretch Intensity:** This workout promotes experimenting with various stretch intensities, giving the quadriceps more depth and variety and allowing for a more customized experience.

8. **Alignment focus:** The Quadriceps Stretch focuses on keeping the body in the proper alignment, encouraging the best possible activation of the core muscles and reducing needless strain.

9. **Dynamic Quadriceps Release:** The stretching motion dynamically releases tension in the quadriceps, which helps one feel empowered and free.

10. **Integration of Strength and Flexibility:** The Pilates repertory benefits significantly from the harmonic integration of strength and flexibility achieved by the Quadriceps Stretch Using Wall.

The Quadriceps Stretch Using Wall becomes a dance in Wall Pilates' elegant choreography, a graceful fusion of strength, flexibility, conscious connection, and precise support. The exercise proves the smooth harmony of the Pilates journey as the quadriceps release smoothly against the wall's soothing embrace. In Pilates, Quadriceps Stretch Using a Wall enables practitioners to transform, creating a harmonious connection between body and soul.

6.7: Cobra Pose with Wall Assistance

In the world of Wall Pilates, the Cobra Pose with Wall Assistance is an enthralling and powerful backbend intended to enhance backbend practice with additional wall assistance. Based on the basic principles of Pilates, this posture smoothly combines the wall's supporting effect with the spine's dynamic extension. Within the Pilates paradigm, the Cobra Pose with Wall Assistance is a transformational exercise that enhances back flexibility, mindful movement, and the development of a strong connection between body and breath.

1. Initial Position:

Starting from an arm's length away from the wall, face the wall to create the Cobra Pose with Wall Assistance. Place both hands at shoulder height on the wall to maintain a tall and straight posture. The spine is neutral, and the feet are hip-width apart. Starting in this posture creates a base alignment by using the wall as a guide to assist the next backbend.

2. Core Engagement and Alignment:

When doing the Cobra Pose, ensure your shoulders are relaxed, and your arms are straight. To maintain the spine and stabilize the pelvis, contract your core muscles. Preventing needless strain and encouraging regulated movement through the back are made possible by the alignment and core engagement, which pave the way for the dynamic expansion of the spine.

3. Intense Backbend Motion:

The dynamic backward extension of the spine is the key to the Cobra Pose with Wall Assistance. The wall offers crucial stability and balance support, enabling a slow and steady movement in the backbend. The spine is purposefully arched during the extension, giving the impression of opening up and stretching. Because the wall acts as constant guidance, backbend practitioners may explore the depth of their flexibility with control and more accuracy.

4. Breathing in Time with Movement:

With wall assistance, breath becomes an essential component of the Cobra Pose. As you prepare for the backbend, take a deep breath and let your rib cage stretch. As you exhale entirely, contract your abdominal muscles and arch your back. Inspiring a mindful Pilates practice and strengthening the link between breath and the therapeutic backbend, the coordinated breath and movement improve awareness.

5. Balance and Alignment Wall Support:

The wall is an essential component of the Cobra Pose, helping to maintain alignment and balance. A point of contact is provided by the hands resting on the wall, which enables a slow and deliberate advancement in the backbend. Without sacrificing stability, the wall takes on a comforting role, allowing practitioners to concentrate on the quality of the stretching exercise.

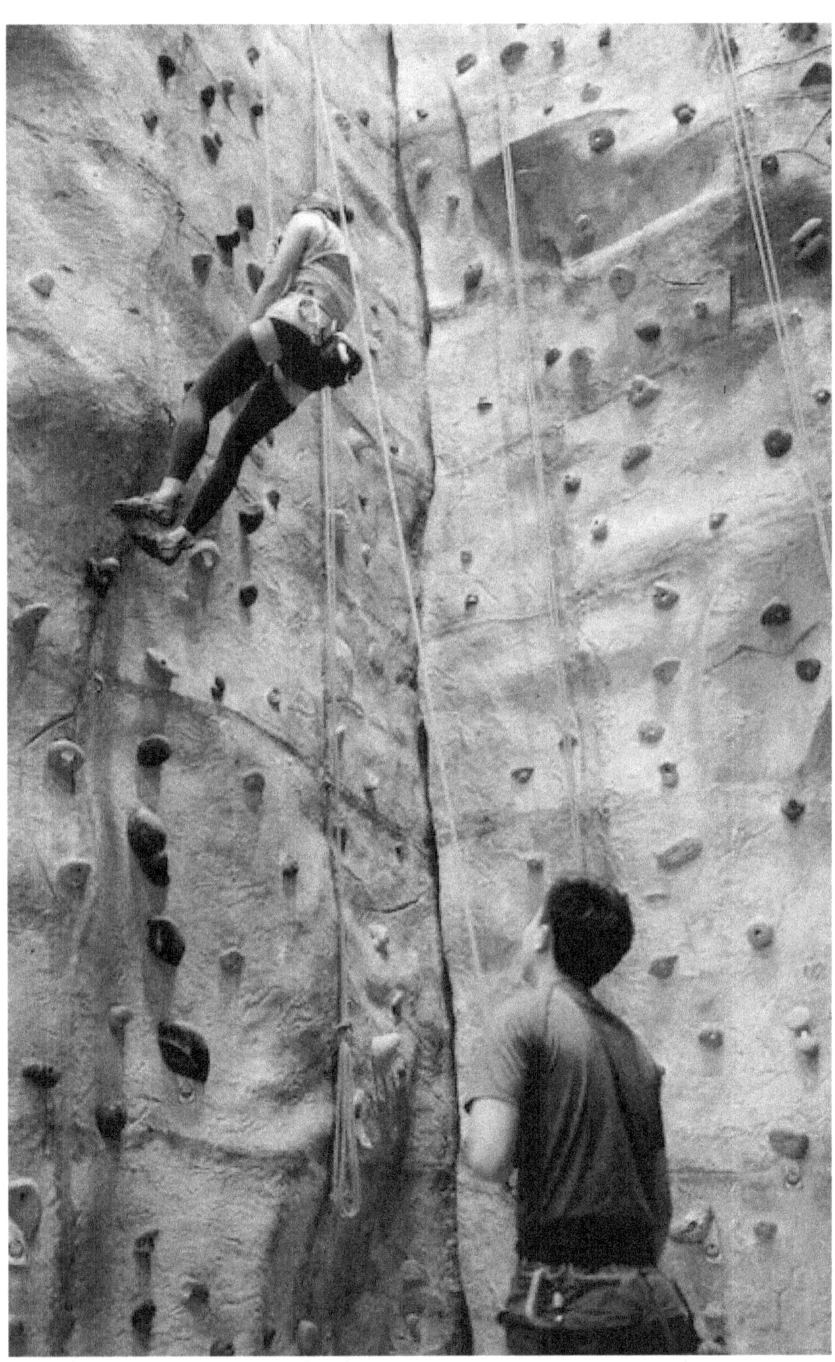

6. Paying Attention to Spinal Extension:

Put your whole attention on the Cobra Pose's spinal extension. As you explore the backbend's depth, notice the back's progressive arching. By improving the mind-muscle link, this cognitive awareness makes it possible to feel spinal flexibility more purposefully and intentionally.

7. Difference in Depth of Backbend:

Experiment with different backbend depths to customize the experience to your comfort level and aspirations. The stretch's intensity may be varied by varying the distance from the wall. Every variant offers a chance for a dynamic and customized experience by bringing subtlety to the backend.

8. Alignment Verification and Adjustment:

Check your alignment from time to time in the Cobra Pose to ensure your arms are straight and your backbend movement stays controlled. Adjustments may be made to suit different comfort levels by varying the distance from the wall. The focus is on achieving a freeing and revitalizing controlled and flowing backbend.

9. Mindful Backbending and Core Engagement: To stabilize the spine in the Cobra Pose, engage your core muscles. By consciously engaging the core, one may have a mindful back-bending sensation that balances strength and release. By including core activation, Pilates encourages a comprehensive approach to spinal flexibility and introduces a therapeutic component to the practice.

10. Smooth Shift and Recuperation:

After completing the Cobra Pose, gently return to the neutral spine posture, taking a deep breath to recognize the extension. Take a deliberate step forward and enjoy your newly acquired flexibility in your back. The recovery phase is a crucial element that highlights the significance of intentional recovery and the dynamic challenge. This thoughtful ending enhances the exercise's overall coherence and efficacy.

Cobra Pose with Wall Assistance Benefits:

1. **Spinal Flexibility Enhancement**: This exercise improves and refines the spine's flexibility, which makes it possible to release stress in a controlled and dynamic manner.

2. **Core Engagement and Stability:** During the dynamic backbend, the Cobra Pose aggressively engages and increases core engagement, which helps to provide general stability and support.

3. **Breath-Movement Synchronization:** This technique adds to a mindful Pilates practice by promoting awareness and maintaining the Cobra Pose's flexibility.

4. **Wall Support for Balance and Alignment:** Through the wall, practitioners may concentrate on the quality of the stretching action while still preserving balance and alignment during the backbend.

5. **Mind-Body Connection:** A deliberate concentration on spinal extension develops a more open and controlled feeling of mind-body awareness within the practice.

6. **Adaptable for Varied Flexibility Levels:** The Cobra Pose with Wall Assistance is flexible, accommodating alterations to suit varying degrees of flexibility and offering opportunities for more complex tasks.

7. **Difference in Backbend Depth:** This practice promotes experimenting with various backbend depths, which adds complexity and variety to the spinal stretch and fosters an individualized experience.

8. **Alignment Emphasis:** The Cobra Pose emphasizes the importance of preserving appropriate alignment, encouraging the best possible activation of the core muscles, and avoiding needless strain.

9. **Dynamic Spinal Extension:** The backbend exercise lengthens and strengthens the spine in a dynamic way, which helps one feel empowered and free.

10. **Synthesis of Strength and Flexibility:** A valuable addition to the Pilates repertory, Cobra Pose with Wall Assistance accomplishes a harmonic synthesis of strength and flexibility.

The Cobra Pose with Wall Assistance becomes a dance in Wall Pilates' elegant choreography, a graceful fusion of power, flexibility, conscious connection, and precise support. The exercise becomes a testimonial to the flawless harmony in the Pilates journey as the spine arches gently against the wall's welcoming embrace. In the domain of Pilates, Cobra Pose with Wall Assistance enables practitioners to go on a transformational journey, creating a harmonious connection between body and soul.

Conclusion

As we end "Wall Pilates Power: A Woman's Guide to Strength and Grace," we reflect on the transforming adventure we've taken together with a feeling of satisfaction and empowerment. This carefully designed manual, intended to support women in their Pilates journey, invites you to experience the balance between grace, strength, and conscious movement in the context of Wall Pilates.

We have explored Pilates's rich history and tenants across the chapters, revealing the knowledge that serves as the cornerstone of this life-changing discipline. We've looked at the many advantages designed especially for women, realizing that the female body's strength and elegance combine to produce a potent combination.

A safe and fulfilling practice has been made possible by the careful arrangement of your Wall Pilates studio, the focus on safety and body awareness, and the fundamentals of stance and posture. Breath rhythm has taken on the role of a friend, assisting you in every action and helping you develop a close relationship with your body and its potential.

Our journey through exercises for balance and stability, flexibility development, spine and posture alignment, upper and lower body toning, and core strengthening has been like a dance. This choreography reveals your inner beauty and resiliency. Every exercise, from simple postures to complex methods, has served as a stepping stone to help you become more conscious of the power and potential in your body.

The practice's use of relaxation and mindfulness recognizes the holistic aspect of well-being. After a workout, the calming exercises and light stretches create a loving environment for physical and emotional healing. As you participate in these mindful exercises, remember that self-care is an essential rather than a luxury—a means of achieving long-term well-being.

You've taken on difficulties in the advanced methods, opening up new avenues for strength and flexibility. These methods are not only physical achievements; they are turning points in your path that demonstrate your tenacity and will.

The book ends with a reminder that Wall Pilates has advantages outside the gym. It is a comprehensive approach that supports mental and physical well-being. Feel the power and elegance resonating within you as you stand in Wall-Assisted Savasana, absorbing the essence of your practice. This exercise celebrates your path towards a harmonious and powerful self and is a testament to your perseverance.

I hope the lessons you find in these pages will never stop inspiring you and leading you to a life full of grace, power, and conscious movement. May the principles of Wall Pilates serve as a continual reminder that your body is a powerful instrument and that your soul is an unwavering force as you incorporate them into your everyday life. Move gracefully, embrace your inner power, and develop an awareness-based relationship with your unique self.

Cheers to the path that never ends—where grace, strength, and deliberate movement become enduring allies, guiding you toward a future in which every stride is a dance and every breath is conscious. Every moment is a chance for personal development.

References

- Seadazed. (2021, December 22). *The History of Pilates (& Why You Should Be Doing Pilates!) — LEVEL UP with Laurie.* LEVEL UP With Laurie. https://www.levelupwithlaurie.com/blog/the-history-of-pilates-why-you-should-be-doing-pilates#:~:text=Pilates%20is%20a%20fitness%20system,of%20the%20mind%2Dbody%20connection.

- *10 Tips for Parents to Teach Children about Body Safety and Boundaries.* (n.d.). https://www.aap.org/en/news-room/news-releases/health--safety-tips/10-tips-for-parents-to-teach-children-about-body-safety-and-boundaries/#:~:text=Discuss%20how%20it%20is%20 never,solid%20 rule%20about%20 inappropriate%20 touches.

- Smith, R. (2023, January 5). *How to breathe in Pilates.* Complete Pilates. https://complete-pilates.co.uk/breathing/

- Bedosky, L. (2023, August 9). *How to do standing leg raises.* BODi. https://www.beachbodyondemand.com/blog/standing-leg-raise

- CPT, C. S., & CPT, A. E. M. (2022, August 24). How to do the wall sit exercise to light up your quads and work your core. *SELF.* https://www.self.com/story/wall-sit-exercise#:~:text=Stand%20with%20your%20back%20against,completely%20pressed%20against%20the%20wall.

- *Adductor / Adduction Inner Thigh Machine – WorkoutLabs exercise guide.* (n.d.). WorkoutLabs. https://workoutlabs.com/exercise-guide/thigh-adductor-inner-thigh-machine/

- Nasm, B. W. (2021, November 2). No cheating allowed with this brutal biceps pump. *Men's Health*. https://www.menshealth.com/fitness/a26142874/biceps-workout-cheat-free/

- *How to do Wall Arm Circles*. (n.d.). [Video]. skimble.com. https://www.skimble.com/exercises/84995-wall-arm-circles-how-to-do-exercise

- *Forward fold against wall yoga (Uttanasana against wall) | Yoga sequences, benefits, variations, and Sanskrit Pronunciation | Tummee.com*. (2019, April 17). Tummee.com. https://www.tummee.com/yoga-poses/forward-fold-against-wall

- Pt, K. G. (2021, May 31). *How to do the supported standing figure 4 stretch*. LIVESTRONG.COM. https://www.livestrong.com/article/13764466-supported-standing-figure-four-stretch/